An Atlas of Investigation and Management
PAEDIATRIC RESPIRATORY DISEASE
AIRWAYS AND INFECTION

An Atlas of Investigation and Management

PAEDIATRIC RESPIRATORY DISEASE

AIRWAYS AND INFECTION

Edited by

Andrew Bush, MB BS(Hons), MA, MD, FRCP, FRCPCH

Professor of Paediatric Respirology and Consultant Paediatric Chest Physician
Department of Paediatric Respiratory Medicine
Imperial College and Royal Brompton and Harefield NHS Foundation Trust
London, UK

Jane C. Davies, MB ChB, MRCP, MRCPCH, MD(Hons)

Reader and Honorary Consultant
Department of Paediatric Respiratory Medicine
Royal Brompton and Harefield NHS Foundation Trust and Imperial College
London, UK

CLINICAL PUBLISHING

OXFORD

Clinical Publishing
an imprint of Atlas Medical Publishing Ltd
Oxford Centre for Innovation
Mill Street, Oxford OX2 0JX, UK

Tel: +44 1865 811116
Fax: +44 1865 251550
Email: info@clinicalpublishing.co.uk
Web: www.clinicalpublishing.co.uk

Distributed in USA and Canada by:
Clinical Publishing
30 Amberwood Parkway
Ashland OH 44805, USA

Tel: 800-247-6553 (toll free within US and Canada)
Fax: 419-281-6883
Email: order@bookmasters.com

Distributed in UK and Rest of World by:
Marston Book Services Ltd
PO Box 269
Abingdon
Oxon OX14 4YN, UK

Tel: +44 1235 465500
Fax: +44 1235 465555
Email: trade.orders@marston.co.uk

A catalogue record for this book is available from the British Library

ISBN-13   978 1 904392 97 2
ISBN e-book   978 1 84692 615 0

Project manager: Gavin Smith, GPS Publishing Solutions, Herts, UK
Illustrations by Graeme Chambers, BA(Hons)
Typeset by Phoenix Photosetting, Chatham, Kent, UK
Printed and bound by Marston Book Services Ltd, Abingdon, Oxon, UK

Contents

Contributors

Ian M. Balfour-Lynn, BSc, MBBS, MD, FRCP, FRCPCH, FRCS(Ed), DHMSA
Consultant in Paediatric Respiratory Medicine
Department of Paediatric Respiratory Medicine
Royal Brompton and Harefield NHS Foundation Trust
London
UK

Siobhán B. Carr, MBBS, FRCPCH, MSc
Paediatric Respiratory Consultant
Department of Paediatric Respiratory Medicine
Barts and The London Children's Hospital
London
UK

Mark A. Chilvers, BSc, MB ChB, MD, MRCPCH
Respiratory Paediatrician
Division of Paediatric Respiratory Medicine
BC Children's Hospital
Vancouver
Canada

Jane C. Davies, MB ChB, MRCP, MRCPCH, MD(Hons)
Reader and Honorary Consultant
Department of Paediatric Respiratory Medicine
Royal Brompton and Harefield Foundation Trust and
Imperial College
London
UK

Fiona Dickinson, MBChB, MRCP, FRCR
Consultant Paediatric Radiologist
Department of Imaging
Leicester Royal Infirmary
Leicester
UK

Julian T. Forton, MRCPCH, PhD
Consultant in Paediatric Respiratory Medicine
The Children's Hospital For Wales
Cardiff
UK

Andrew R. Gennery, MD, MRCP, FRCPCH, DCH
Reader/Honorary Consultant in Paediatric Immunology
and HSCT
Institute of Cellular Medicine
Child Health
University of Newcastle upon Tyne
UK

Jonny Harcourt, MA (Oxon), FRCS
Consultant Otolaryngologist
Department of Paediatric Otolaryngology
The Chelsea and Westminster and Royal Brompton
Hospitals
London
UK

Albert M. Li, BSc, MBBch, MD, MRCPCH, MRCP(UK), FHKCP, FHKAM (Paed)
Professor and Honorary Consultant Paediatrician
Department of Paediatrics
Prince of Wales Hospital
The Chinese University of Hong Kong
Shatin
Hong Kong

Indra Narang, BMedSci, MBBCH, FRCPCH, MD
Consultant Respirologist
Division of Respiratory Medicine
Hospital for Sick Children
Toronto, Ontario
Canada

Chris O'Callaghan, BMedSci, FRCP, FRCPCH, DM, PhD
Professor of Paediatrics
Division of Child Health and Institute of Lung Health
Department of Infection, Immunity and Inflammation
University of Leicester
Leicester
UK

David Anthony Spencer, MB BS (Hons), MD, MRCP, FRCPCH
Consultant in Respiratory Paediatrics
Department of Respiratory Paediatrics and Cystic Fibrosis
Great North Children's Hospital
Newcastle upon Tyne Hospitals NHS Foundation Trust
Newcastle upon Tyne
UK

Ranjan Suri, MBChB, MRCPCH, MD
Paediatric Respiratory Consultant and Honorary Senior
Lecturer
Department of Respiratory Paediatrics
Great Ormond Street Hospital for Children
Portex Unit
UCL Institute of Child Health
London, UK

Anne H. Thomson, MD, FRCP, FRCPCH
Consultant in Paediatric Respiratory Medicine
Oxford Children's Hospital
The John Radcliffe
Oxford
UK

Abbreviations

ADA	adenosine deaminase
AHI	apnoea hypopnoea index
AI	apnoea index
AR	autosomal recessive
ASL	airway surface liquid
ATP	adenosine triphosphate
BCG	Bacillus Calmette-Guérin
BiPAP	bi-level positive airway pressure
BTS	British Thoracic Society
CaCC	calcium-activated chloride channel
CF	cystic fibrosis
CFTR	cystic fibrosis transmembrane conductance regulator
CgC	common interleukin g chain
CHARGE	Coloboma of the iris and retina, Heart disease, Atresia of choanae, Retarded growth, Genital hyperplasia, Ear defects
COPD	chronic obstructive pulmonary disease
CPAP	continuous positive airway pressure
CSA	central sleep apnoea
DIOS	distal intestinal obstruction syndrome
ENaC	epithelial sodium channel
ENT	ear, nose and throat
FBC	full blood count
FEV_1	forced expiratory volume in one second
FiO_2	fraction of inspired oxygen
FVC	forced vital capacity
GOR	gastro-oesophageal reflux
GP	general practitioner
HDU	high dependency unit
HiB	*Haemophilus influenzae* type B
HIV	human immunodeficiency virus
hMPV	human metapneumovirus
HRCT	high-resolution computed tomography
IF	immunofluorescence
Ig	immunoglobulin
IL-7Ra	interleukin 7 receptor a
JAK-3	janus-associated kinase 3
MBL	mannose-binding lectin
MCC	mucociliary clearance
MDR TB	multidrug-resistant tuberculosis
MRSA	Methicillin-resistant *Staphylococcus aureus*
NICE	National Institue for Health and Clinical Excellence
NO	nitric oxide
OAI	obstructive apnoea index
OME	otitis media with effusion
ORCC	outwardly rectifying Cl⁻ channel
OSAS	obstructive sleep apnoea syndrome
$PaCO_2$	arterial carbon dioxide tension
PCR	polymerase chain reaction
PEFR	peak expiratory flow rate
PICU	paediatric intensive care unit
PJP	*Pneumocystis jiroveci* pneumonia
PPI	proton pump inhibitors
PSG	polysomnography
RAG	recombination activating genes
RAST	radioallergosorbent test
RSV	respiratory syncytial virus
SaO_2	arterial oxygen saturation
SCID	severe combined immunodeficiency
TB	tuberculosis
URTI	upper respiratory tract infection
WCC	white cell count
XL	X-linked
ZAP-70	zeta-associated kinase-70

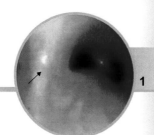

Chapter 1

Asthma: diagnosis and assessment

Ian M. Balfour-Lynn

Introduction

Childhood asthma and recurrent viral wheezing are two of the most common conditions that general practitioners (GPs) and paediatricians assess and treat. Despite concerns that asthma has been becoming more common worldwide, it seems that visits to GPs and hospital admissions for asthma have been reducing over the last decade in children aged less than 14 years (**1.1**). Nevertheless, prevalence is approximately 10% and over half of all cases of asthma begin in childhood. This chapter covers diagnosis and assessment (**1.2**) but treatment has not been included (the

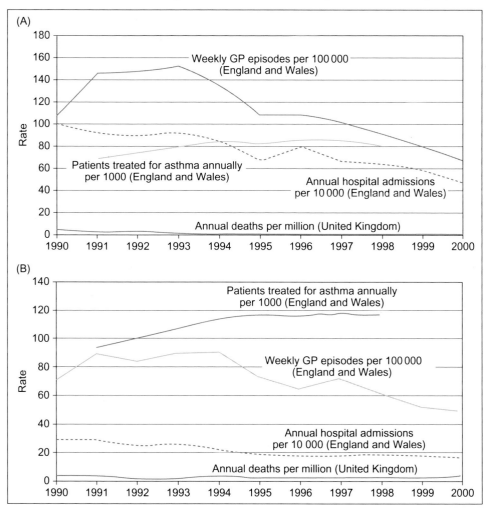

1.1 Trends in annual rates for primary care consultations, hospital admissions and mortality for asthma among children aged <5 years (A) and aged 5–14 years (B). Taken from Gupta R, Strachan D. Asthma and allergic diseases. In: *The Health of Children and Young People*. Office for National Statistics, March 2004. Available from: *www.statistics.gov.uk/children/*.

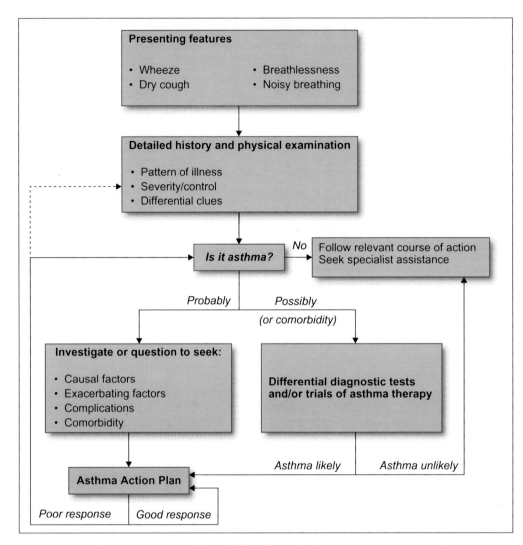

1.2 Diagnosis of asthma in children (from: BTS/SIGN guideline on the management of asthma. *Thorax* 2003; 58(Suppl 1): i1–i94).

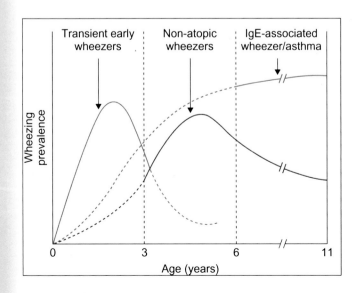

1.3 Hypothetical yearly peak prevalence of wheezing for three different wheezing phenotypes in childhood. The dashed lines suggest wheezing can present different curve shapes due to many different factors, including overlap of the groups. Reproduced with permission from Stein RT, Holberg CJ, Morgan WJ, *et al*. Peak flow variability, methacholine responsiveness and atopy as markers for detecting different wheezing phenotypes in childhood. *Thorax* 1997; 52: 946–52.

UK guidelines can be consulted for details of the stepwise approach to treatment).

Recurrent wheezing in infancy is nearly always associated with viral upper respiratory tract infections. There is a reluctance to give an infant under 2 years of age the label of 'asthma'; however, features suggesting the child has genuine infantile asthma include personal and family history of atopy and a pattern of cough/wheeze whereby symptoms are more chronic than episodic. The diagnosis of asthma becomes more obvious as the child gets older and continues to have recurrent cough and wheeze.

Three different wheezing phenotypes have been identified in the first 11 years of life (**1.3**). The group of 'transient early wheezers' tends to have reduced lung function that persists through childhood. The 'non-atopic wheezers' of infants, toddlers and early school years are mostly associated with increased peak flow variability, which may persist long after the wheezing itself ceases. The third group is IgE-associated wheeze/asthma, which may occur at any stage during childhood and is related to a combination of atopy, increased bronchial responsiveness and increased peak flow variability.

History

The history is critical in making the diagnosis and is often the only factor that can be relied upon. It is important to realize there is confusion among parents as to what is meant by wheeze, and the harsh sounds made by upper airway secretions are often mistaken for wheeze. Specific pointers to asthma are outlined in *Table 1.1*.

The differential diagnosis of recurrent wheeze is quite large (*Table 1.2*). Points suggesting alternative diagnoses are shown in *Table 1.3* and, in particular, symptoms that started in the first weeks of life, and particularly on the first day of life, need careful diagnostic evaluation.

Examination

Examination of the child is often unremarkable. Attention needs to be paid to growth, chest shape and auscultation. Chest shape may reveal bilateral Harrison sulci or an increased anterior–posterior diameter, which can indicate frequent or chronic airways obstruction (**1.4**). Auscultation may well be normal at the time in a clinic setting; however, asthma should be suspected if wheeze is heard by a health

Table 1.1 Symptoms and other points in history suggestive of asthma	
Cough	Recurrent
	Dry, tight
	Non-productive
	Night-time
	Exercise-induced
	Not always/only with viral URTIs
	Onset usually after 3–4 months of age
Wheeze (assuming there really is a wheeze)	Recurrent
	Exercise-related
	Associated with furry household pets
	Induced by viral URTIs
Breathlessness or difficulty breathing	Particularly shortly after onset of exercise and relieved by rest
Other symptoms	Otherwise well child, i.e. no other symptoms, normal growth
Risk factors	Past history, e.g. premature birth, mechanical ventilation, bronchiolitis requiring hospitalization.
	Signs of atopy, e.g. atopic eczema, hay fever, genuine food allergy, particularly to egg
Family history	Parents or siblings with asthma, eczema, hay fever
	Smoking parents

URTI, upper respiratory tract infection.

professional and distinguished from upper airway noises. If the child is acutely unwell, there may be wheeze, tachypnoea, recession and even cyanosis. Beware the silent chest with inadequate air entry, which indicates severe bronchospasm and is an emergency. Part of the examination must include watching how the child takes their inhaled medication. This is often done poorly and it is critical to ensure the child has an age-appropriate device, which is undamaged and being used correctly.

Table 1.2 Non-asthmatic causes of wheeze (or noises that may be mistaken for wheeze)

Upper airway disease	Adenotonsillar hypertrophy, rhinosinusitis, postnasal drip
Congenital structural airway disease	Complete cartilage rings, cysts, webs
Bronchial/tracheal compression	Vascular rings and sling, enlarged cardiac chamber, lymph nodes enlarged by tuberculosis or lymphoma, congenital thoracic malformations
Endobronchial disease	Foreign body, tumour
Oesophageal/ swallowing problems	Gastro-oesophageal reflux, incoordinate swallow, laryngeal cleft or H-type tracheo-oesophageal fistula
Chronic pulmonary suppuration	Cystic fibrosis, primary ciliary dyskinesia, immunodeficiency, bronchiectasis of unknown aetiology
Miscellaneous	Obliterative bronchiolitis, bronchopulmonary dysplasia, congenital or acquired tracheo/bronchomalacia, pulmonary oedema

Table 1.3 Points in the history suggesting alternative diagnosis

- What the child/family are describing is not really wheeze
- Upper airway symptoms: snoring, constant rhinitis, sinusitis
- Symptoms from the first days of life
- Very sudden onset of symptoms
- Chronic moist cough or sputum production
- Wheeze associated with feeding, irritable after feed, worse lying down, vomiting
- Choking on feeds
- Any feature of a systemic immunodeficiency
- Chronic diarrhoea, poor growth
- Disappearance of symptoms when asleep

Table 1.4 Points in the examination suggesting alternative diagnosis

- Digital clubbing
- Signs of weight loss, failure to thrive
- Upper airway disease: enlarged tonsils and adenoids, prominent rhinitis, nasal polyps
- Severe chest deformity out of proportion to symptoms
- Fixed monophonic wheeze
- Stridor (monophasic or biphasic)
- Asymmetric wheeze (louder or restricted to one side)
- Signs of cardiac or systemic disease

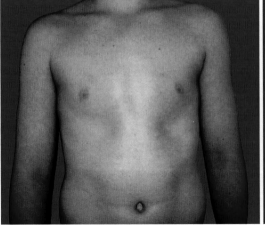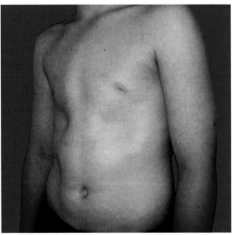

1.4 Marked chest deformity with Harrison sulci in a 12-year-old steroid-dependent asthmatic boy.

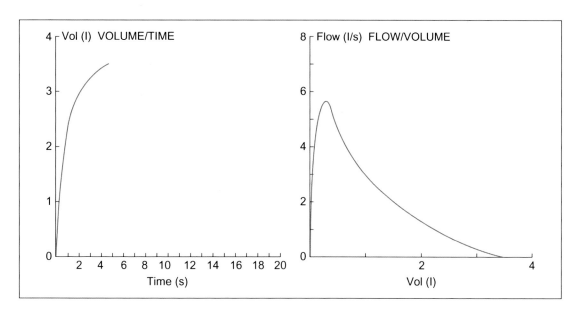

1.5 Spirometric flow volume loop in a 16-year-old asthmatic girl, indicating mild obstructive airways disease likely to be due to asthma. The forced expiratory volume in 1 second was 67% and forced vital capacity 103% predicted.

Certain features are strongly suggestive of an alternative diagnosis to asthma (*Table 1.4*).

Investigation to confirm diagnosis

No single investigation can give 100% confirmation of asthma, which is essentially a clinical diagnosis. However, some simple tests will strengthen the likelihood of the diagnosis, such as measurement of peak expiratory flow rate. Measurement of flow volume loops with spirometry can give even more information than simple peak flow rates. Spirometry may show an obstructive pattern on the flow-volume loop, with greater reduction in forced expiratory volume in 1 second than forced vital capacity (**1.5**). If a bronchodilator is then given, repeat spirometry may indicate the degree of bronchodilator responsiveness (**1.6**). Spirometry before and after exercise may also reveal exercise-induced bronchospasm. Skin-prick testing for common aeroallergens (e.g. grass and tree pollens, house dust mite, aspergillus mould, cat and dog) will indicate atopic status (**1.7**). A chest radiograph may exclude several diagnoses and may show hyperinflation in more severe cases (**1.8**). Response to anti-asthma therapy can be very useful for confirming the diagnosis.

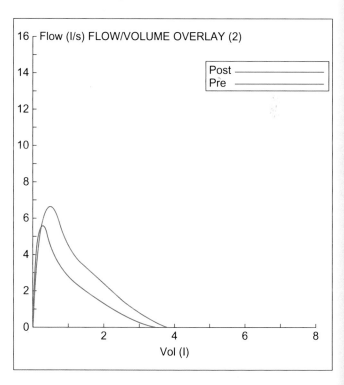

1.6 Spirometric flow volume loop pre-bronchodilator (green) and post-bronchodilator (red) in a 16-year-old asthmatic girl, showing a 19% absolute rise in percentage predicted forced expiratory volume in 1 second, i.e. a moderate degree of bronchodilator responsiveness.

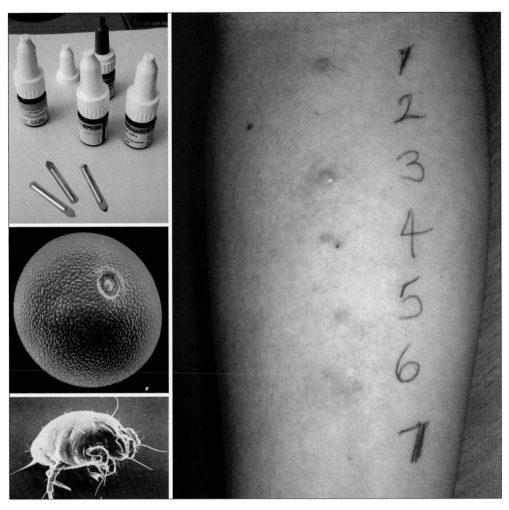

1.7 Skin-prick testing in an asthmatic child who was mildly positive to dog (no. 5), more positive to grass pollen (no. 3) and strongly positive to house dust mite (no. 6). He was not allergic to cat (no. 4) or aspergillus mould (no. 7). Positive histamine control (no. 1) and negative control (no. 2) are also done. Also shown are some of the allergen solutions and lancets used for the test; grass pollen and a house dust mite – *Dermatophagoides pteronyssinus* (not to scale).

Further investigations may be required to exclude alternative and concomitant diagnoses (*Table 1.5*), most of which are covered in detail in other chapters of this atlas.

Assessment of asthma severity

History should include the impact on school attendance, disturbed sleep, hospital admissions, courses of oral corticosteroids, and the dose of inhaled corticosteroids required to stay symptom-free. Examination may reveal Harrison's sulci and hyperinflation. Lung function may be surprisingly normal, even in those with severe chronic asthma. A peak flow meter can also be used at home, and if measured once or twice daily over a period of a week or so, marked peak flow variability can indicate poor control.

Assessment of difficult asthma

Referral of a child with apparently severe asthma to a tertiary unit requires a complete and systematic re-evaluation of the situation. The commonest reasons for failure to respond to asthma treatment are that the treatment is not being taken

Table 1.5 Investigations specific for alternative diagnoses

Diagnosis	Investigations
Gastro-oesophageal reflux	pH study, isotope milk scan
Vascular ring	Chest radiograph, spirometry, flexible bronchoscopy, echocardiography, barium swallow, HRCT angiography
Vocal cord dysfunction	Spirometry, laryngoscopy
Cystic fibrosis	Sweat test, stool elastase, DNA analysis
Inhaled foreign body	Expiratory chest radiograph, rigid bronchoscopy
Obliterative bronchiolitis	HRCT chest scan, adenovirus titres in serum
Bronchiectasis	HRCT chest scan
Primary ciliary dyskinesia	Nasal ciliary brushings, nasal nitric oxide
Tracheo/bronchomalacia	Flexible bronchoscopy, bronchography
Recurrent aspiration	Bronchoalveolar lavage for lipid-laden macrophages, chest X-ray, HRCT chest scan, video fluoroscopy
Immune deficiency	Immune function testing

HRCT, high-resolution computed tomography.

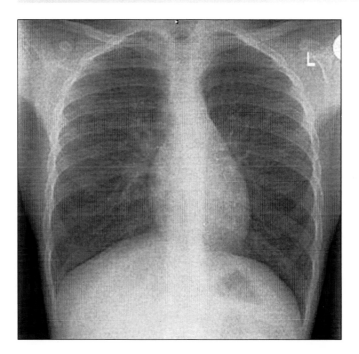

1.8 Chest radiograph of an 8-year-old asthmatic boy, showing hyperinflation.

Step 1
- Allergy testing
- Spirometry and reversibility
- Chest radiograph
- Sweat test
- Salivary cotinine
- Exhaled nitric oxide (NO)
- ± Prednisolone, cortisol, theophylline blood levels

- Respiratory nurse specialist home visit
- Detailed history including psychosocial, environmental exposure
- Assess inhaler technique
- Contact local hospital regarding accident and emergency visits and admissions
- Contact GP, chemist regarding prescription usage
- Contact school regarding medication policy, absence

1.9 Step 1 of the Royal Brompton Hospital protocol for assessment of children with difficult asthma.

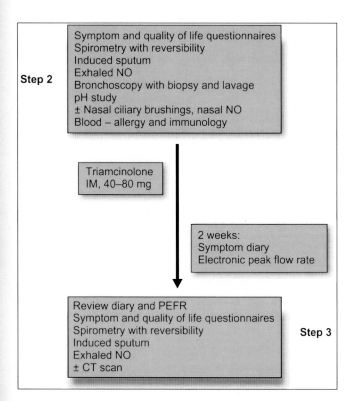

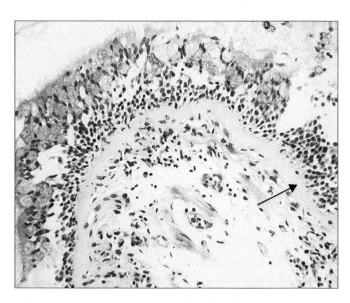

1.12 Endobronchial biopsy in a child with difficult asthma showing inflammation and a thickened reticular basement membrane (arrow).

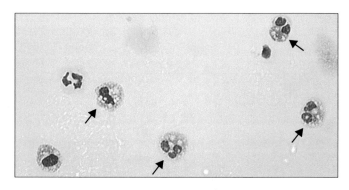

1.13 Induced sputum from an asthmatic patient showing predominance of eosinophils (arrows). Stained with diffquik, 40× magnification (courtesy of G. Nicholson).

1.10 Steps 2 and 3 of the Royal Brompton Hospital protocol for assessment of children with difficult asthma. During step 2 assessment, intramuscular triamcinolone is given at the time of the bronchoscopy and step 3 takes place 2 weeks later.

or that the child does not have asthma. The diagnostic approach undertaken at the Royal Brompton Hospital for children with difficult asthma is outlined in **1.9** and **1.10**. The inflammatory cell profile from an endobronchial biopsy or induced sputum may help direct further treatment (**1.11–1.13**).

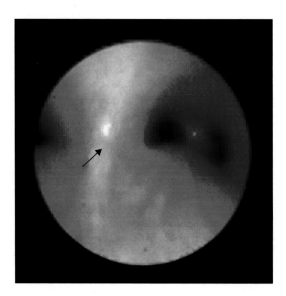

1.11 Flexible bronchoscopy at the level of the carina (arrow) showing macroscopic severe inflammation in a 5-year-old with difficult asthma.

Further reading

British Thoracic Society, Scottish Intercollegiate Guidelines Network. British guideline on the management of asthma. *Thorax* 2008; 63(Suppl iv): iv1–iv121.

Gupta R, Strachan D. Asthma and allergic diseases. In: *The Health of Children and Young People*. Office for National Statistics, March 2004. Available from: *www.statistics. gov.uk/children/*.

Payne DNR, Balfour-Lynn IM. Difficult asthma in children: a practical approach. *J Asthma* 2001; 38: 189–203.

Saglani S, Nicholson AG, Scallan M, *et al*. Investigation of young children with severe recurrent wheeze: any clinical benefit? *Eur Respir J* 2006; 27: 29–35.

Stein RT, Holberg CJ, Morgan WJ, *et al*. Peak flow variability, methacholine responsiveness and atopy as markers for detecting different wheezing phenotypes in childhood. *Thorax* 1997; 52: 946–52.

Chapter 2

Diseases of the upper airway

Jonny Harcourt

Introduction

Paediatric otolaryngology provides care for diseases of the upper airways. This includes middle ear, nose and sinus disease as well as management of the paediatric airways.

The majority of consultations in general paediatric otolaryngology involve either hearing loss (and speech delay), recurrent ear and upper airway infections as well as breathing problems particularly sleep-disordered breathing.

Ear

The commonest form of paediatric ear disease is otitis media with effusion (OME) (**2.1**) and/or recurrent acute otitis media, which may be a frequent complication of OME. The natural history of the condition is spontaneous improvement. An acute episode can be complicated by acute

mastoiditis (**2.2**); this is where the purulent process breaks out of the middle ear cleft and extends under the periosteum of the mastoid bone, producing an egg-like swelling behind the ear, which pushes the pinna forward. It is a surgical emergency as the infective process may also be spreading inwards towards the intracranial compartment. An urgent mastoidectomy is required.

OME can be treated by correcting any nasal disease contributing to eustachian tube dysfunction but in the majority of children the principal decision is to whether ventilation tube (grommet) insertion is merited. This is considered in children who have persistent bilateral significant conductive hearing loss that is producing an observable delay in speech and social development. The placement of ventilation tubes should normalize the hearing but requires a general anaesthetic in a child and leaves the ear vulnerable to infection passing in through the grommet while washing or swimming. A residual perforation after

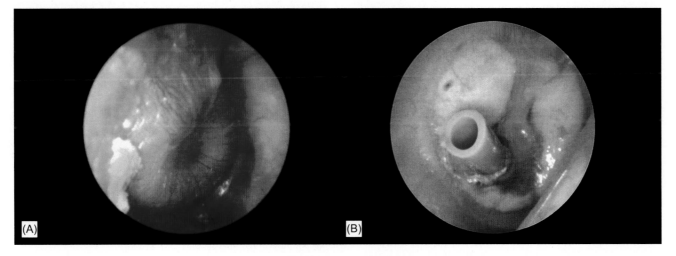

2.1 Otitis media with effusion. (A) Eustachian tube dysfunction leads to a chronic mucoid middle ear effusion, which may produce a conductive hearing loss and encourage bouts of acute otitis media. (B) Ventilation tube re-aerating the middle ear.

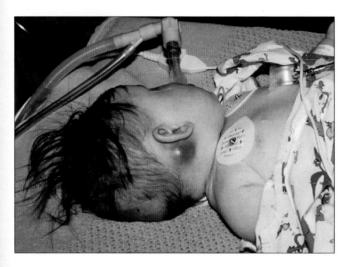

2.2 Acute mastoiditis. Secondary to acute otitis media, pus escapes from the middle ear cleft under the soft tissues under the retro-auricular area pushing the pinna forwards. A surgical emergency because of the associated risk of meningitis.

extrusion of the ventilation tube is possible and OME may reoccur once the middle ear ventilation is once more dependent on the eustachian tube.

Chronic otitis media remains a rare condition in children in the Western world and is due either to recurrent or chronic infection of a tympanic membrane perforation or

due to the development of a non-toileting retraction pocket (cholesteatoma) (**2.3**). This expansile and lytic disease can cause middle ear and temporal bone damage as well as act as the nidus for intracranial sepsis. It requires tympanomastoid surgery to control the disease.

Congenital or rapidly progressive hereditary sensorineural hearing loss occurs in about 1:1000 births (the majority are non-syndromic). In the UK it is screened for by neonatal oto-acoustic emission testing. This has led to early detection of affected individuals with the possibility of optimum auditory rehabilitation, including cochlear implantation that has the potential of giving children open-set hearing.

Nose and sinuses

Choanal atresia is an uncommon congenital abnormality, which is due to a failure of the nasal cavity to cannalize posteriorly in to the nasopharynx (**2.4**). It may be part of a CHARGE association (**C**oloboma of the iris and retina, **H**eart disease, **A**tresia of choanae, **R**etarded growth, **G**enital hypoplasia, **E**ar defects). If bilateral, then it causes severe respiratory distress at birth as neonates are obligatory nasal breathers. The airway can be stabilized by an oral airway until definitive surgery is carried out.

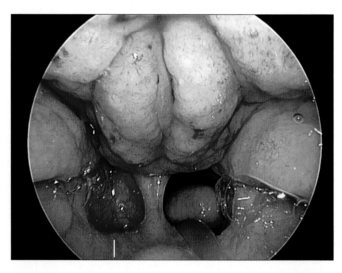

2.4 Unilateral choanal atresia. View from nasopharynx looking forward. The left posterior choana is atretic (arrow), while the right is patent. The adenoids are prominent. Often, such cases are only diagnosed in infancy, whereas bilateral choanal atresia causes acute breathing problems at birth.

2.3 Cholesteatoma. Chronic dysfunction in the tympanic cavity, particularly in the attic region, leads to a retraction in which squamous debris collects, shed from the epithelial surface of the retraction. The process extends causing erosive damage to the middle ear and leading to chronic otorrhoea and occasionally to serious infective complications such as a cerebral abscess.

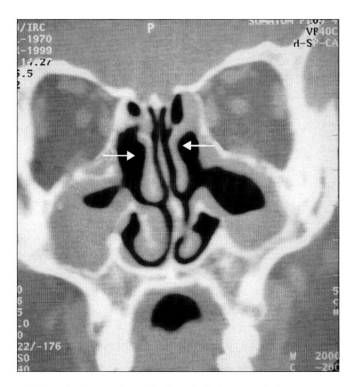

2.5 Chronic sinusitis in cystic fibrosis. This computed tomography scan of the sinuses shows the typical findings in cystic fibrosis of small or absent frontal sinuses, deficient lateral nasal wall even without previous surgery, and sinus mucosal thickening.

Nasal obstruction in children is often due to adenoidal hypertrophy. The presence of a large adenoidal pad in the nasopharynx disrupts the natural mucus drainage from the nasal cavity and leads to pooling of nasal secretions and persistent rhinorrhoea. It also encourages acute or chronic infection. The adenoids atrophy after 5 years of age and so many of these symptoms may resolve with conservative management but, in the presence of severe symptoms, an adenoidectomy may be justified.

Chronic nasal symptoms may raise the possibility of sinobronchial disease such as primary ciliary dyskinesia or cystic fibrosis (**2.5**). In the latter, nasal polyps are very frequent but in the former, despite disordered mucociliary clearance, they are rare. Unilateral mucopurulent nasal discharge is very suggestive of a nasal foreign body and this diagnosis should be considered until proved otherwise.

Sinus disease is very rare before adolescence, as the paranasal sinuses are very rudimentary in infancy though acute maxillary sinusitis may occur in neonates. In adolescence, as with adults, acute or chronic rhinosinusitis, particularly of the ethmoid and frontal sinuses, can lead to a periorbital cellulitis, which requires urgent management because of the risk of ischaemic blindness (**2.6**).

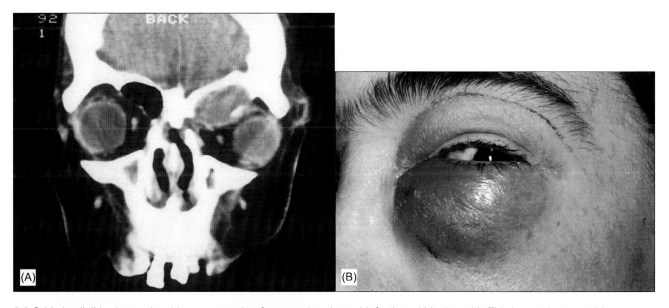

(A)

(B)

2.6 Orbital cellulitis. Acute sinusitis can spread to form a subperiosteal infection within the orbit. This is a serious condition with the risk of ischaemic visual loss and an orbital abscess. Urgent orbital decompression may be necessary. (A) Computed tomography scan showing proptosis and subperiosteal collection. (B) Orbital cellulitis in early stages. The edges of the cellulitis have been marked.

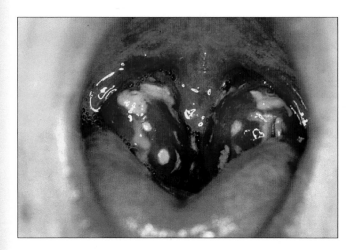

2.7 Acute follicular tonsillitis. Enlarged tonsils with follicular purulent eruption.

Tonsils and oral cavity

Recurrent upper airway infections in children are usually caused by viral infections with the hallmarks of seasonality and widespread symptoms (nasal obstruction, sore throat and cough). Recurrent bacterial tonsillitis is rare before the age of 5 and if present has a good chance of spontaneous improvement by school-age. To justify a tonsillectomy, recurrent tonsillitis should occur at least six times in a calendar year, or four or more times per year in two consecutive years. Each episode should be associated with systemic upset and evidence of acute bacterial infection, including significant pain, cervical lymphadenopathy, anorexia and persistence over more than 3 days (**2.7**). The recovery period for the surgery is 2 weeks and there are small risks of reactionary and secondary haemorrhage. An alternative diagnosis to consider with any acute pharyngitis is glandular fever for which reason amoxicillin is avoided as an antibiotic treatment (**2.8**).

Obstructive sleep apnoea is a commoner indication for adeno-tonsillectomy in the pre-school age group due to tonsillar (**2.9**, see also Chapter 3) and/or adenoidal hypertrophy. General anaesthesia in children with obstructive sleep apnoea may be challenging; great care is required to manage the airway in the immediate postoperative period due to the risk of obstruction, and in children under 15 kg with complex medical problems or obesity; this may mean a short stay on an HDU or PICU.

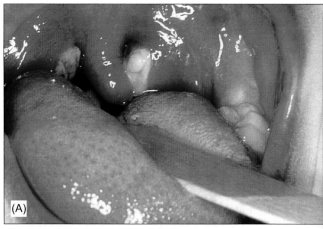

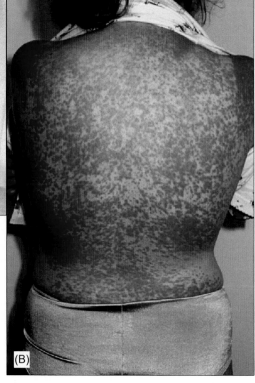

2.8 Glandular fever. (A) Slough over tonsils generalized pharyngitis and involving the soft palate. (B) Widespread papular rash erupting after treatment with amoxicillin of patient with glandular fever.

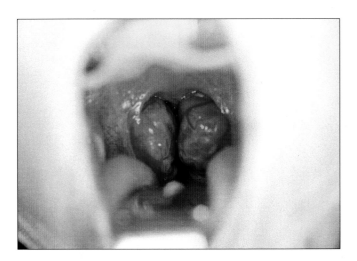

2.9 Tonsillar hypertrophy. Enlarged tonsils, even in the absence of acute or chronic infection may cause obstructive sleep apnoea, particularly in the infant group.

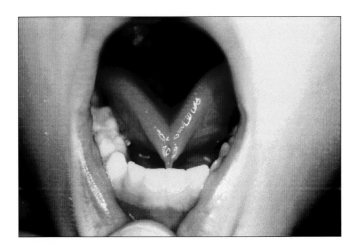

2.10 Tongue tie. A tight tongue frenulum that may cause suckling problems in the newborn or dysarthria in infants.

A common oral abnormality is a tongue tie (**2.10**). The tongue frenulum should be considered for release if it is causing problems with infant feeding or speech.

Larynx and trachea

Specialist paediatric otolaryngology services are often based around the management of stridor. This high-pitched breathy sound is indicative of airway obstruction beyond the pharynx; turbulent air movement in this section of the airway produces stertor, a low-frequency sound, a form of which is snoring. The relevant part of the respiratory cycle when stridor occurs may suggest the level of obstruction. Inspiratory sounds are usually due to narrowing at the supraglottic or glottic levels (above or at the level of the vocal cords). Biphasic stridor is usually due to obstruction in the subglottis or extrathoracic trachea and expiratory stridor due to intrathoracic problems. The severity of the obstruction can be gauged by the inspiratory effort and use of extrathoracic muscles, as well as pallor, pulse, respiratory rate and failure to thrive. Outpatient assessment of patients with stridor may be achieved with flexible endoscopy either in clinic or at the bedside, but the optimal diagnostic procedure is a micro-laryngoscopy and bronchoscopy performed under general anaesthesia but with the child spontaneously ventilating. This allows an excellent dynamic view of the airway and the performance of therapeutic interventions such as laser excision, stent insertion or removal of obstructing secretions or a foreign body.

The commonest cause of neonatal stridor is laryngomalacia (**2.11**). This is a misnomer as there is no abnormality of the laryngeal cartilage but a variation of the anatomy of the larynx with tight vertical aryepiglottic folds with prominent cuneiform cartilages and an 'omega'-shaped epiglottis. For the majority of cases, it is purely a matter

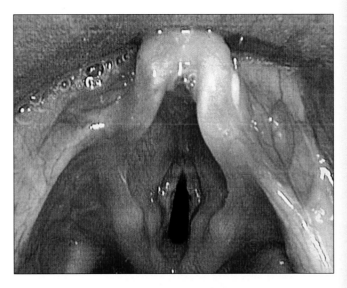

2.11 Laryngomalacia. Omega-shaped epiglottis with prominent corniculate cartilages in the aryepiglottic folds. This causes dynamic collapse during inspiration and stridor, often when feeding.

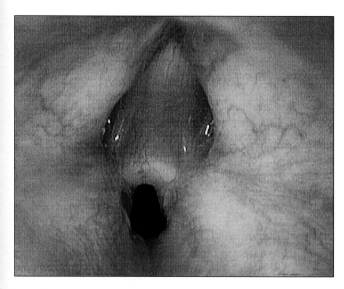

2.12 Glottic web. Occasionally membranous, but usually part of anterior subglottic stenosis. May be part of velo-cardio-facial syndrome (22q11.2 deletion).

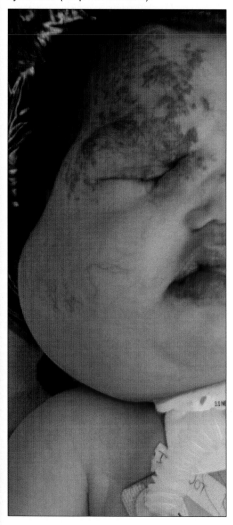

2.14 Laryngeal cysts. (A) Supraglottic congenital saccular cyst (differential diagnosis would be a laryngocoele or cystic hygroma). (B) Subglottic cysts are common in neonates who have been intubated for a prolonged period.

2.13 Neonatal head and neck haemangioma causing airway obstruction. Extensive haemangiomas can cause progressive airway obstruction until spontaneous involution. May occur in the subglottis, usually in the posterolateral position.

of reassurance once the diagnosis has been made with a flexible endoscope. The symptoms disappear within the first 2 years of life with no long-term functional implication. In a minority of neonates, there is a failure to grow due to the severity of the condition and an association with severe acid reflux secondary to strong respiratory effort, particularly during feeding. In such cases, an aryepiglottoplasty is an effective procedure to reduce the supraglottic collapse during inspiration by reducing the bulk of the aryepiglottic folds. This can be done by laser or scissors dissection during a micro-laryngoscopy and bronchoscopy.

Other uncommon congenital problems include a glottic web (**2.12**), which usually requires an open repair. Capillary haemangiomas (**2.13**) may cause airway obstruction either by their extensive size or predilection to forming in the subglottis. There is a variety of philosophies of management depending on whether an attempt is made to clear the airway of the vascular lesion or to bypass the obstruction with a tracheostomy (while awaiting the eventual involution of the lesion). The latter is best avoided if possible due to the risks of secondary scarring in the airway though endoscopic or open removal of haemangiomas can also cause airway compromise. Laryngeal clefts are also rare but may be missed during routine endoscopic assessments of the airway. If large, they produce severe problems, but if limited to the larynx, they may present with recurrent aspiration and go unnoticed unless the inter-arytenoid area is probed during endoscopy.

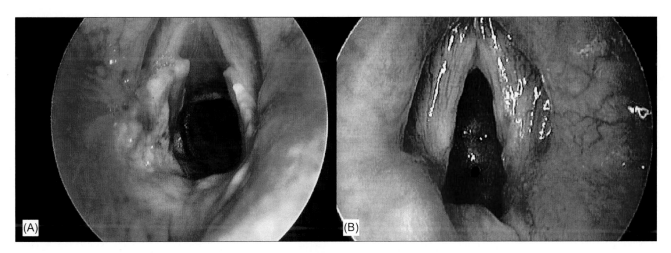

(A) (B)

2.15 Subglottic stenosis. (A) Post-intubation trauma to the posterior larynx. (B) Pinhole airway following development of severe subglottic stenosis.

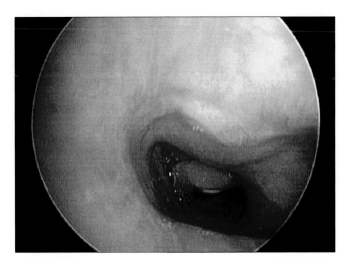

2.16 Suprastomal granulation and collapse. Endoscopic picture of upper trachea above an *in situ* tracheostomy. There has been mild secondary tracheal wall collapse and granulation as a result of the long-term presence of the tube.

Laryngeal cysts may be part of a large congenital abnormality or be secondary to prolonged intubation and are usually managed with laser resection (**2.14**).

The management of subglottic stenosis (**2.15**) is a large subject in itself and is beyond the scope of this chapter but it is important to state that the best form of treatment is prevention. If a tracheostomy is formed to avoid prolonged intubation then it may also lead on to chronic airway problems such as suprastomal collapse and granulation (**2.16**), which may make decannulation difficult or dangerous.

Airway infections of interest include recurrent respiratory papillomatosis (**2.17**), which is due to human papillomavirus 6 and 11 probably transmitted to a child during vaginal delivery of an infected mother. It is a condition that spontaneously involutes after 10 years of age and the management is also of symptom control by debulking the disease in the larynx (and trachea if very extensive) using

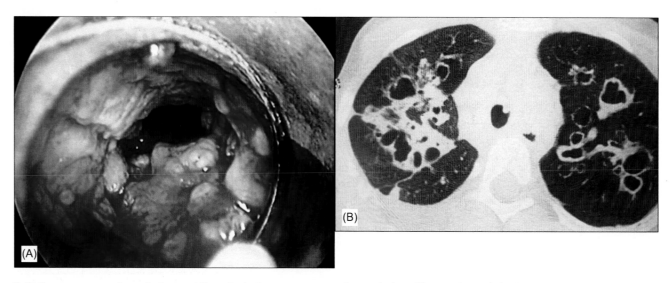

2.17 Severe recurrent respiratory papillomatosis. In severe cases airway viral papillomas due to infection with human papillomavirus 6 and 11 spread beyond the larynx to involve (A) the trachea and bronchi and (B) the lung parenchyma causing bullae formation.

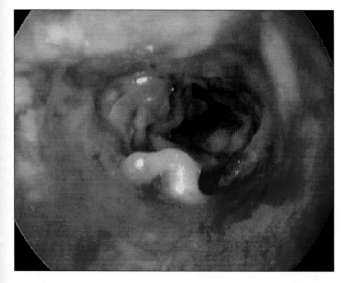

2.18 Acute bacterial tracheitis. Staphylococcal infection of the trachea in an adolescent with production of copious occluding mucopurulent secretions.

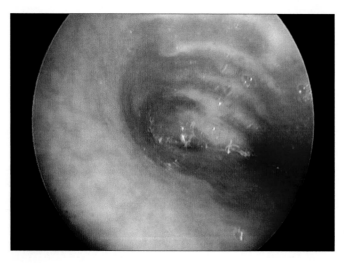

2.19 Tracheomalacia. Distal tracheal collapse may be either primary with congenital abnormalities of the tracheal cartilage (often associated with vascular abnormalities) or secondary to local inflammation or trauma from cardiac or oesophageal surgery or disease.

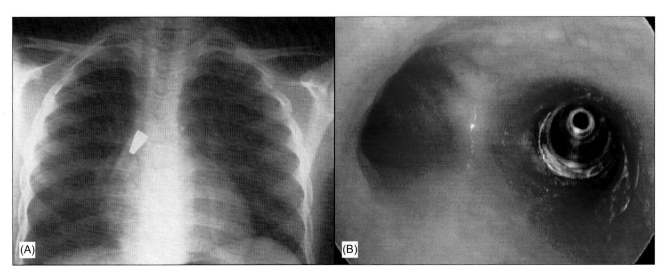

2.20 Metallic airway foreign body. (A) Chest X-ray showing foreign body in the right main bronchus. (B) Rigid bronchoscopic picture of pen top in right main bronchus.

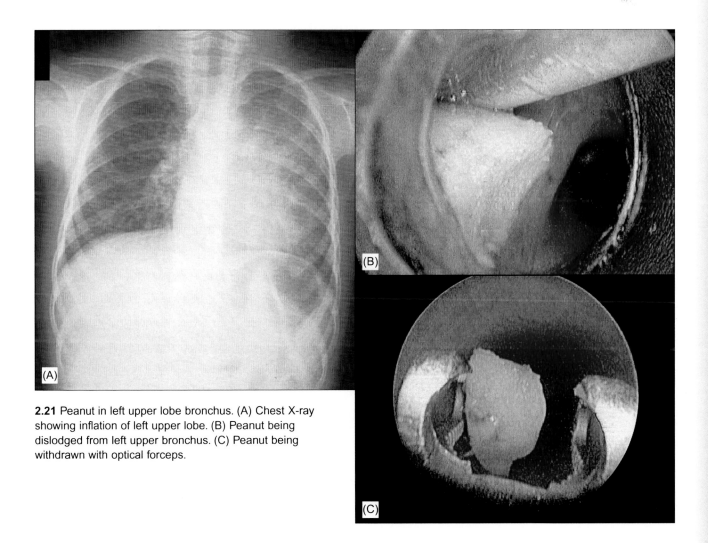

2.21 Peanut in left upper lobe bronchus. (A) Chest X-ray showing inflation of left upper lobe. (B) Peanut being dislodged from left upper bronchus. (C) Peanut being withdrawn with optical forceps.

a laser or micro-debrider while awaiting spontaneous improvement. Acute bacterial tracheitis (**2.18**) is a rare condition of older children due to staphylococcal infection causing massive mucopurulent collection within the main airways and for which an emergency micro-laryngoscopy and bronchoscopy may be life saving.

Tracheomalacia (**2.19**) is due to abnormalities of the tracheal rings that are either congenitally short, leading to worsening airway collapse with respiratory effort, or become softened secondary to other local disease such as a tracheo-oesophageal fistula or its surgical treatment. Patients may suffer 'dying spells' with severe dyspnoea and cyanosis leading to collapse and sudden recovery. Surgical treatment may be necessary either to excise the affected portion of the trachea or to stent with either a tracheostomy tube or a tracheal stent.

Airway foreign bodies may be managed by either rigid or flexible bronchoscopy (**2.20, 2.21**) and a balanced approach is necessary, which may require close co-operation between paediatric otolaryngology and respiratory medicine.

Further reading

Cotton R, Myer C. *Practical Pediatric Otolaryngology*. Philadelphia: Lippincott-Raven, 1999.

Harcourt J. Congenital abnormalities of the upper airway. In: *Kendig's Disorders of the Respiratory Tract in Children*. Chernick V, Boat TF, Wilmott RW, Bush A (eds). Philadelphia: Saunders Elsevier, 2006, pp. 288–95.

Chapter 3

Sleep-disordered breathing in children

Albert M. Li

Introduction

Sleep-disordered breathing is increasingly being recognized as an important disease entity and if the underlying condition is left untreated then significant morbidity and even mortality can result. The most prominent sleep-disordered breathing in children is obstructive sleep apnoea syndrome (OSAS), which belongs to the severe end of a spectrum, ranging from the frank, intermittent occlusion seen in OSAS, to persistent, primary snoring. This chapter will mainly concentrate on the epidemiology, diagnosis and management of OSAS.

Obstructive sleep apnoea syndrome

OSAS in children is characterized by repeated episodes of partial or complete upper airway obstruction during sleep that result in disruption of normal ventilation and sleep patterns. Prompt recognition and institution of treatment has a tremendous impact on child healthcare as OSAS may produce serious cardiovascular and neurocognitive consequences.

Epidemiology

Published studies utilising different diagnostic cutoffs have yielded different prevalence rates. The condition peaks between the age of 2 and 8 years (*Table 3.1*), coinciding with the peak age of lymphoid hyperplasia. It has an equal gender distribution in prepubertal children, but an increased prevalence in boys after puberty. Children of African American origin, with a positive family history, and those with chronic upper and lower respiratory diseases are at higher risk.

Aetiology

Adenotonsillar hypertrophy is the commonest cause, although this alone cannot account for the pathophysiological process. There is accumulating evidence to suggest that OSAS is related to an interaction of structural and neuromuscular variables within the upper airway. Patients do not obstruct their airway during wakefulness. Some patients with no other known risk factors have persistent OSAS despite having their tonsils and adenoids removed. The mechanism appears related to a combination of three processes:

1. decreased upper airway patency (adenotonsillar hypertrophy, allergies associated with chronic rhinitis or nasal obstruction);
2. reduced capacity to maintain airway patency related to neuromuscular tone (obesity, neuromuscular disorder), and;
3. decreased drive to breathe (brainstem).

A variety of medical conditions are associated with increased risk (*Table 3.2*, **3.1–3.3**). Since its first description in 1976, childhood OSAS has been recognized as a very different disease entity from adult OSAS with respect to aetiology, clinical manifestations and management (*Table 3.3*).

Clinical features

The commonest presenting complaint is snoring; the condition is unlikely in the absence of habitual snoring (most nights), although most snoring children do not have OSAS. *Table 3.4* outlines associated symptoms. In a study of 50 children, confirmed as OSAS at the author's unit, the frequency of different presenting features is tabulated in **3.4**.

Table 3.1 Prevalence of childhood OSAS

Author	Year of publication	Number of subjects	Country	Age (years)	Diagnostic technique	Prevalence of OSAS
Ali (*Arch Dis Child* 1993; 68: 360–6)	1993	782 screened 132 monitored	UK	4–5	Pulse oximetry, video	0.7%
Gislason (*Chest* 1995; 107: 963–6)	1995	454	Iceland	0.5–6	PSG (AHI >3)	2.9%
Redline (*AJRCCM* 1999; 159: 1529–32)	1999	126	USA	2–18	PSG	1.6% (AHI >10) 10.3% (AHI >5)
Brunetti (*Chest* 2001; 120: 1930–35)	2001	895 screened 12 monitored	Italy	3–11	PSG (AHI >3)	1.8%
Anuntaseree (*Pediatr Pulmonol* 2001; 32: 222–7)	2001	1142 screened 8 monitored	Thailand	6–13	PSG (AHI >1)	0.69%
Castronovo (*J Pediatr* 2003; 142: 377–82)	2003	595 screened 265 monitored	Italy	3–6	Pulse oximetry	13%
Rosen (*J Pediatr* 2003; 142: 383–9)	2003	243	USA	8–11	PSG (OAI >1)	1.9%

AHI, apnoea–hypopnoea index; OAI, obstructive apnoea index; OSAS, obstructive sleep apnoea syndrome; PSG, polysomnographic study.

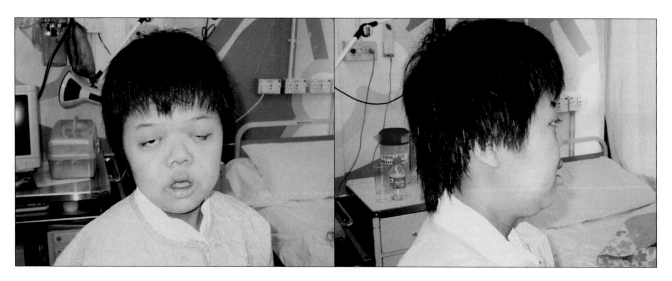

3.1 Child with Crouzon's syndrome: note the marked maxillary hypoplasia.

Table 3.2 Medical conditions associated with childhood obstructive sleep apnoea syndrome

Craniofacial syndromes	• Crouzon syndrome • Apert syndrome • Treacher-Collins • Goldenhar syndrome • Pierre Robin syndrome
Neurological diseases	• Arnold–Chiari malformation • Meningomyelocoele • Cerebral palsy • Duchenne muscular dystrophy
Conditions with abnormal muscle tone	• Down syndrome • Prader–Willi • Hypothyroidism
Conditions with reduced upper airway patency	• Adenotonsillar hypertrophy • Obesity • Allergic rhinitis • Macroglossia • Laryngomalacia • Subglottic stenosis • Mucopolysaccharidoses/ metabolic storage diseases

Table 3.3 Comparison of obstructive sleep apnoea syndrome in children and adults

	Children	Adults
Estimated prevalence	1–3%	2–4%
Peak age	2–8 years	30–60 years
Gender (M/F)	1:1	8:1
Weight	Normal, decreased, increased	Overweight
Major cause	Adenotonsillar hypertrophy	Obesity
Gas exchange abnormalities	Always	Always
Duration of obstructive apnoeas	Any	>10 seconds
Abnormal AI	>1	>5
Abnormal AHI	>1	>10
Sleep architecture	Preserved	Always altered
Arousals	Occasional	Always
Complications	Poor attention Hyperactivity Hypertension	Hypertension Daytime sleepiness
Treatment of choice	Adenotonsillectomy	CPAP, weight reduction

AHI, apnoea–hypopnoea index; AI, apnoea index; CPAP, continuous positive airway pressure.

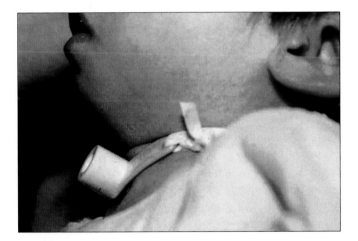

3.2 Child with Pierre Robin syndrome. Note the small chin. In the supine position, the tongue would fall back easily causing upper airway obstruction.

No combination of symptoms and physical findings has been found to reliably distinguish OSAS from primary snoring. In most cases, children have enlarged tonsils (**3.5**) and/or adenoids and they do not demonstrate breathing difficulties during clinical examination. There is no reliable relationship between the size of the tonsils on direct inspection and the presence of OSAS. *Table 3.5* shows the parameters that should be assessed during physical examination of a child with OSAS.

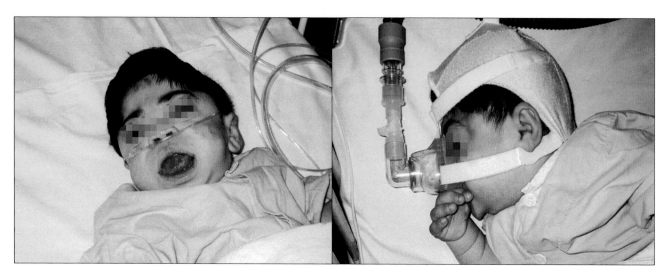

3.3 Child with mucolipidosis type II with excessive accumulation of abnormal tissue in the upper airway causing obstruction. He was started on continuous positive airway pressure for his obstructive sleep apnoea syndrome.

Table 3.4 Symptoms of childhood obstructive sleep apnoea syndrome

Nocturnal symptoms	• Loud habitual snoring • Difficulty breathing when asleep • Apnoeic pauses • Restless sleep • Sweating • Dry mouth • Abnormal sleeping position • Enuresis • Night terrors/sleep walking • Bruxism/teeth grinding
Daytime symptoms	• Mouth breathing • Morning headache • Difficulty waking up • Mood changes • Poor attention span/academic problems • Increased nap/daytime sleepiness • Chronic nasal congestion/ rhinorrhoea • Frequent upper respiratory tract infections • Difficulty swallowing/poor appetite • Hearing problems

Complications associated with obstructive sleep apnoea syndrome

Neurocognitive abnormalities

In contrast to adult patients, affected children tend to have preserved sleep architecture and therefore excessive daytime sleepiness is not usually a predominant feature. However, there is an association with significant behavioural and learning problems, poor attention span, hyperactivity and lower than average IQ, all of which may be reversible with treatment.

Exposure to intermittent hypoxia during the sleep cycle of adult rats is associated with significant spatial learning deficits as well as increased neuronal apoptosis within susceptible brain regions such as the hippocampus and cortex. Grey matter loss within brain regions that have a role in cognitive function has been demonstrated in patients with OSAS, suggesting that altered oxygen homeostasis during sleep causes neural cell loss and consequent neurobehavioural morbidities. Upregulation and activation of several proinflammatory mediators such as platelet-activating factor, excitotoxic glutamate, oxidative products and phospholipids cyclooxygenase-2 could account for the hypoxia-induced spatial deficits seen in rats. Whether the same mechanism applies to humans will need further exploration. There is current evidence to suggest that micro/subcortical arousals could also play a part in neurocognitive dysfunction seen in childhood OSAS.

Table 3.5 Physical examination of a child with obstructive sleep apnoea syndrome

Growth	• Overweight, obesity • Failure to thrive
Facial features	• Adenoidal facies secondary to chronic mouth breathing • Maxillary hypoplasia • Micrognathia • Macroglossia
Evidence of atopy	• Eczema • Features of allergic rhinitis
Evidence of enlarged adenoids and/or chronic nasal congestion	• Mouth breathing • Hyponasal speech • High arched palate
Oropharyngeal examination	• Enlarged tonsils • Overcrowding of teeth
Cardiorespiratory examination	• Chest wall deformity • Evidence of systemic or pulmonary hypertension

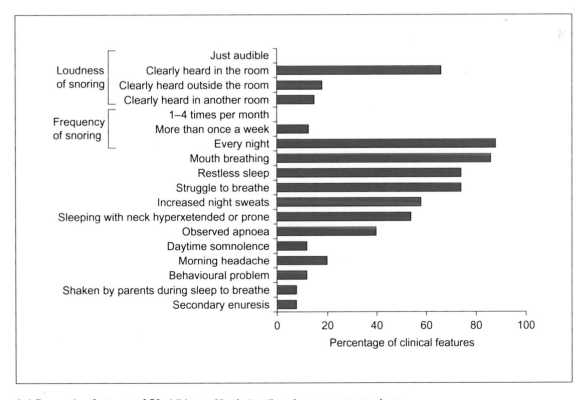

3.4 Presenting features of 50 children with obstructive sleep apnoea syndrome.

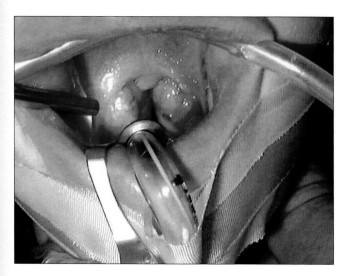

3.5 Enlarged tonsils.

anthropomorphic measurements were taken before and after adenotonsillectomy in 14 children confirmed to have OSAS. Average sleeping energy expenditure decreased, and mean weight Z-score increased postoperatively without any change in caloric intake. The presence of poor appetite, difficulty swallowing and nausea with vomiting were reported more frequently in children with OSAS compared with controls. In a separate study, 60% of children with OSAS were slow eaters and 37% had problems with swallowing. Statistically significant increases in weight and insulin-like growth factor levels were found in a group of OSAS children following adenotonsillectomy. Fortunately, we are seeing less of this complication as parents are becoming more aware of this condition and seeking medical intervention early.

Diagnosis of obstructive sleep apnoea syndrome

Symptoms alone have a poor diagnostic yield. Physical examination is often normal. Currently, the 'gold standard' for the diagnosis of OSAS is overnight polysomnography (PSG) (**3.6, 3.7**). However, normative standards for PSG determination have been chosen on the basis of statistical distribution of data, and it has not been established that those standards have any validity as predictors of long-term outcome. An adaptation effect of the sleep laboratory environment, known as the first-night effect, has been described that disrupts sleep architecture and may lead to an underestimation of respiratory disturbances. Despite the presence of the first-night effect, single-night PSG is adequate and more cost-effective than two consecutive nights in the assessment of childhood OSAS.

Cardiovascular abnormalities

In adults, the presence of OSAS is clearly associated with a risk of systemic hypertension, which reverses with continuous positive airway pressure (CPAP) treatment. Cyclical hypoxia during sleep with alterations in the renin–angiotensin axis and enhanced sympatho-adrenal discharge is being proposed as the underlying mechanism. Decreased right ventricular ejection fraction with abnormal wall motion as well as left ventricular hypertrophy and abnormal geometry have been documented in children with OSAS. Higher diastolic pressures were found in children with OSAS, compared with those with primary snoring. Abnormal blood pressure variability, higher night-to-day systolic pressure ratios and a smaller nocturnal dip in mean blood pressure were documented in a study utilizing 24-hour ambulatory blood pressure monitoring. In the same study, significant association was found between frequency of obstructive apnoeas, oxygen desaturation and arousal with abnormal blood pressure control.

Terminology

- *Obstructive apnoea*: an absence of oronasal airflow in the presence of continued respiratory effort lasting longer than two respiratory cycles (**3.8**).
- *Hypopnoea*: 30–50% reduction in airflow accompanied by hypoxaemia and/or arousal.
- *Central apnoea*: absence of oronasal airflow and respiratory effort lasting for longer than 20 seconds or any duration if accompanied by hypoxaemia (oxygen desaturation of 3% or greater) and/or arousal (**3.9**).
- *Mixed apnoea*: apnoea with both central and obstructive components.
- *Obstructive hypoventilation*: partial airway obstruction leading to: (a) a peak end-tidal CO_2 >55 mmHg or end-tidal CO_2 >45 mmHg for >60% of total sleep time,

Growth failure

The pathogenesis of failure to thrive in children with OSAS is likely to be an interplay between various mechanisms, including increased resting energy expenditure, difficulty with swallowing secondary to enlarged tonsils and abnormal release of growth-related hormones. Caloric intake and sleeping energy expenditure as well as

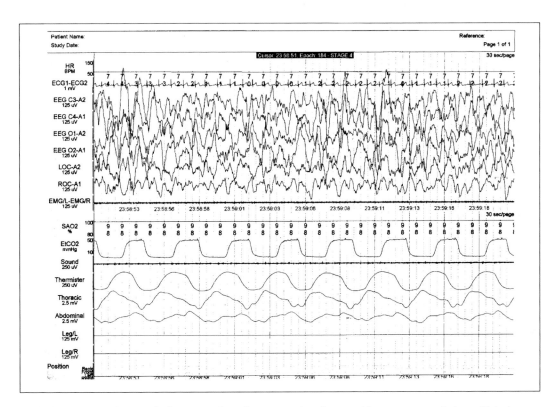

3.6 Polysomnography epoch demonstrating slow wave sleep/non-rapid eye movement sleep. Note large amounts of high amplitude, slow-wave EEG activity.

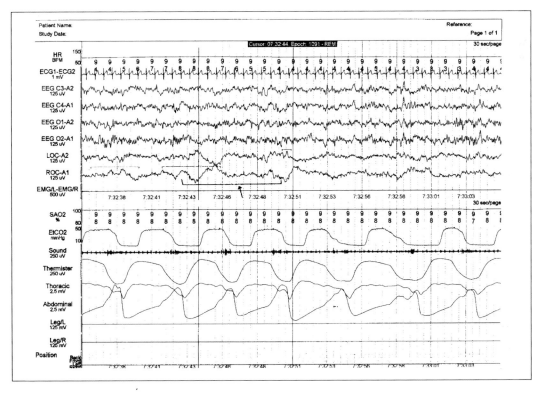

3.7 Polysomnography epoch demonstrating rapid eye movement sleep. Note low voltage EEG activity and episodic rapid eye movements (arrow).

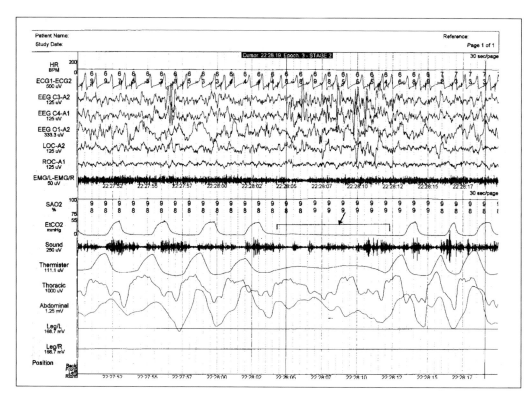

3.8 Polysomnography epoch demonstrating an episode of obstructive apnoea. Note the complete cessation of airflow (arrow).

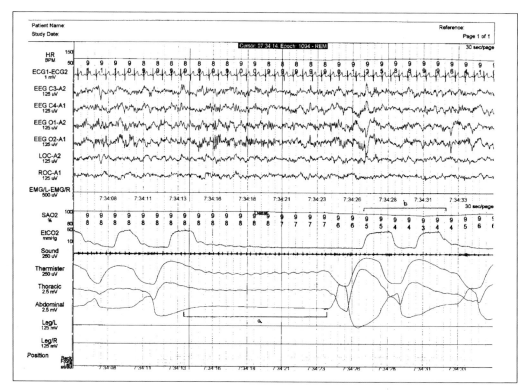

3.9 Polysomnography epoch demonstrating an episode of central apnoea. Note (a) complete cessation of airflow, chest and abdominal movement, and (b) oxygen desaturation following the event.

or (b) end-tidal >55 mmHg for >10% of total sleep time (in the absence of lung disease).

- *Apnoea index*: number of obstructive and central apnoeic events per hour of sleep.
- *Apnoea–hypopnoea index*: number of obstructive and central apnoeic and hypopnoeic events per hour of sleep.

Most paediatric respiratory clinicians consider an obstructive apnoea index >1 to be abnormal. However, this criterion does not take into account episodes of hypopnoea and recently an apnoea–hypopnoea index >1.0 has been proposed as diagnostic for OSAS.

A proper overnight PSG in children should include all the mandatory leads (see below). Tests with incomplete inclusion of these mandatory leads will be categorized as an 'abbreviated study'. The overnight recording should last a minimum of 6 hours, but optimally 8 hours.

The following recording parameters are mandatory (in bold) during PSG:

- **respiratory effort:** chest wall and abdominal motion; this parameter is used to differentiate central from obstructive apnoeas;
- **airflow:** oral and nasal thermisters but the signal is not quantitative; an alternative is the measurement of nasal pressure; this parameter is used to classify cessation of flow into apnoeas or hypopnoeas;
- **heart rate:** electrocardiography;
- **oxygen saturation:** pulse oximeter;
- **sleep stage:** electroencephalogram, usually with two central and two occipital channels;
- **electromyogram of chin;**
- **electro-oculogram;**
- **arousals:** electroencephalogram;
- **leg movements:** anterior tibialis electromyogram;
- **snoring:** microphone; and
- **body positions.**

End-tidal PCO_2 sampling at the nose and/or mouth or transcutaneous CO_2 and video recording are considered optional recording parameters. Some units also measure oesophageal pressure with transoesophageal balloon manometry for the evaluation of upper airway resistance syndrome (its actual existence in children is still being debated) but this is not done routinely. The interpretation of PSG is beyond the scope of this chapter, as it requires considerable experience and detailed examination of the data.

A variety of screening tests have been proposed, including pulse oximetry, audiotaping and radiography. They were all compared with polysomnography as the gold standard with its inherent problems as mentioned above. Most tests were found to have acceptable positive predictive value but less than desirable specificity and negative predictive value.

Who should have a sleep study?

- Those with symptoms suggestive of OSAS should be investigated further. Some would argue that a child with only snoring and without other OSAS symptoms should be investigated.
- Those with an underlying condition that would predispose an individual at a higher risk for OSAS, such as craniofacial anomalies or syndromic diagnosis, for example Down or Prader–Willi syndrome.
- Those who are obese. Obese children are at 10-fold greater risk than normal weight children of suffering from OSAS.

This is very much the author's own personal experience and clinical practice; whether the same guidelines can be followed by others depends on local resources.

Treatment of obstructive sleep apnoea syndrome
Medical treatment
Nasal corticosteroids have recently been examined as an alternative to adenotonsillectomy in otherwise healthy children with OSAS. In a prospective, randomized, double-blinded study, children with mild-to-moderate OSAS were treated with a 6-week course of either nasal corticosteroids or placebo. The authors were able to demonstrate a moderate improvement in cases treated with nasal corticosteroids associated with decreases of 50% in both the desaturation index and the movement arousal index. In contrast, the placebo group did not show any improvement. In an open-labelled study, the leukotriene receptor antagonist montelukast was found to be clinically effective in reducing disease severity in children with mild OSAS.

Surgical treatment
A few studies have provided evidence that adenotonsillectomy is superior to either adenoidectomy or tonsillectomy alone. A recent study reported complete surgical cure of OSAS in about 25% of children while another 50% showed significant improvements in their OSAS parameters. The following groups of patients have been identified to be at

a higher risk for persistent OSAS despite surgery: initial severe OSAS, obesity and those with a positive family history of OSAS. Other surgical procedures such as nasal septoplasty, epiglottoplasty, uvulopharyngopalatoplasty and maxillofacial surgery are seldom performed in children but may be indicated in selected cases.

Mechanical treatment (see also Chapter 6)

Nasal CPAP provides positive pressure to the lumen of the airway, and decreases airway collapsibility. It is of utmost importance that the initial approach to the family and child be performed correctly and successfully. CPAP therapy should be titrated during PSG to determine effective pressures. Children on CPAP treatment should be followed regularly to ensure compliance and proper fit of the mask interface. CPAP may be indicated in the following clinical situations.

- Adenotonsillectomy not indicated or contraindicated.
- Adenotonsillectomy fails to completely resolve symptoms, usually in children with additional risk factors such as obesity.
- Before surgery in children with severe OSAS.

Bi-level positive airway pressure (BiPAP) also allows the setting of a backup rate, and provides some ventilatory assistance. This is particularly important for patients with sleep-related hypoventilation caused by muscle weakness, neurological disease or obesity.

Both CPAP and BiPAP are highly efficacious in paediatric obstructive apnoea but treatment is associated with a high dropout rate. One potential complication of long-term nasal mask CPAP or BiPAP is mid-face hypoplasia. In children on long-term nasal positive pressure therapy, maxillomandibular growth should be monitored carefully and regularly.

Even though our understanding and knowledge of childhood OSAS has expanded exponentially over the last few years, there remain many unanswered diagnostic and mechanistic questions. Recent evidence indicates that childhood OSAS cannot be easily classified into simple clinical entities. The associated symptoms in children may vary and may be difficult to detect. The diagnosis of the condition in children is not straightforward, with the use of polysomnography in separating snoring children into categories being a gross simplification. Further advancement in this important field of paediatric medicine can only be made with international collaborative research utilizing evidence-based definitions, standardized techniques and diagnostic criteria. Further research work should give a better insight into the origins of adult morbidity resulting from childhood sleep-related breathing problems and how it can be prevented.

Central cause of sleep-disordered breathing

Central sleep apnoea (CSA) is rare in children. It occurs in patients with a variety of lower brainstem lesions. The brainstem controls breathing, thus any disease or injury affecting this area may result in problems with normal breathing during sleep or when awake. Conditions that can cause central sleep apnoea include encephalitis affecting the brainstem, congenital anomalies such as Chiari malformation (3.10), neurodegenerative illnesses, and stroke affecting the brainstem. Other causes include complications of surgery of the cervical spine, secondary to radiation in the region of the cervical spine, severe degenerative changes in the cervical spine and/or base of skull, or primary alveolar hypoventilation syndrome.

CSA may also result from disorders such as strokes, heart failure and kidney failure, which can interfere with the brain's control of breathing. People with CSA experience repeated, prolonged periods of apnoea during sleep, often followed by periods of rapid breathing (Cheyne–Stokes breathing). This pattern repeats itself throughout the night. In CSA, the airway remains open, but the signals controlling respiratory muscles are not regulated properly. This causes wide fluctuations in the level of carbon dioxide in the blood. CSA happens during sleep because when a person is awake breathing is usually stimulated by other signals, including conscious awareness of breathing rate.

Primary alveolar hypoventilation syndrome (Ondine's curse) is a congenital central hypoventilation syndrome due to a disorder in the autonomic control of breathing in the absence of any primary disease. Although the incidence is low, it may be underestimated due to the variable clinical expression of this syndrome. Early diagnosis is of great importance to provide appropriate management to prevent the acute and chronic asphyxia that determines the long-term prognosis of this disease. Genetic mutation has recently been identified for this condition.

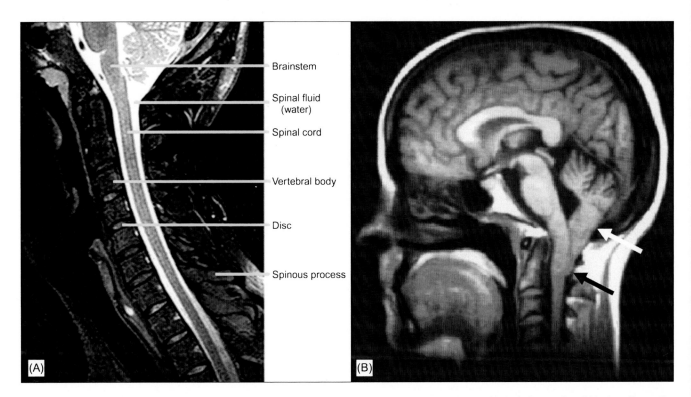

Brainstem

Spinal fluid (water)

Spinal cord

Vertebral body

Disc

Spinous process

(A)

(B)

3.10 Magnetic resonance imaging of the brain and cervical spine provide the most accurate method of diagnosing Chiari malformation. (A) Normal sagittal view of upper cervical cord. (B) Note the descent of the inferior vermis and cerebellar hemispheres through the foramen magnum with a displacement of the brainstem (arrows).

Further reading

American Thoracic Society. Standards and indications for cardiopulmonary sleep studies in children. *Am J Respir Crit Care Med* 1996; 153: 866–78.

Halbower AC, Mahone EM. Neuropsychological morbidity linked to childhood sleep-disordered breathing. *Sleep Med Rev* 2006; 10: 97–107.

Lipton AJ, Gozal D. Treatment of obstructive sleep apnea in children: do we really know how? *Sleep Med Rev* 2003; 7:61–80.

Maitra A, Shine J, Henderson J, Fleming P. The investigation and care of children with congenital central hypoventilation syndrome. *Cur Paediatr* 2004; 14: 354–60.

Rechtschaffen A, Kales A. *A manual of standardized terminology, techniques and scoring system for sleep stages of human subjects*. Brain Information Service/Brain Research Institute, University of California, Los Angeles, California 90024.

Section on Pediatric Pulmonology, Subcommittee on Obstructive Sleep Apnea Syndrome. American Academy of Pediatrics. Clinical practice guideline: diagnosis and management of childhood sleep apnea syndrome. *Pediatrics* 2002; 109:704–12.

Virtual Symposium – Adult and Pediatric Sleep-disordered Breathing. *Proc ATS* 2008; 5: 242–74.

Chapter 4

Lower respiratory tract infection in the normal host

Julian T. Forton, Anne H. Thomson

Introduction

Lower respiratory tract infections are common in children. The majority are viral in aetiology and occur in infants and children under the age of 5 years. In this chapter, we consider bronchiolitis, pneumonia, parapneumonic disease, lung abscess and sequelae of lower respiratory tract infection in the normal host.

Bronchiolitis

Bronchiolitis is the term used to describe viral lower respiratory infection presenting with cough, tachypnoea and recession in infants and young children. Diffuse fine crackles are heard on auscultation.

Aetiology

Respiratory syncytial virus (RSV) is the major cause. In temperate climates, RSV disease occurs in annual winter epidemics. Most infants are infected in their first year of life, and 40% develop lower respiratory tract symptoms. Between 1% and 3% develop severe disease requiring hospital treatment. This results in an estimated 20 000 admissions annually in the UK.

Other viruses that cause bronchiolitis include adenovirus, parainfluenza virus 1, 2 and 3, and influenza virus A and B. Human metapneumovirus (hMPV), discovered in 2001, causes similar disease. In a recent 25-year study from the USA, 20% of previously virus-negative lower respiratory infections were positive for hMPV, implicating hMPV in 12% of all lower respiratory infections.

Clinical features

The majority of children with bronchiolitis present between 2 and 6 months of age. The infant initially presents with coryzal symptoms, a low-grade fever and a cough. This is followed by dyspnoea, which increases over the next few days. Infants are tachypnoeic with recession and hyperinflation and possibly hypoxia. Auscultation reveals fine, scattered crackles, prolonged expiration and often, expiratory wheeze. Very young or preterm infants may present with apnoea.

Radiological features

Chest X-ray is not routinely performed; findings are non-specific, with hyperinflation and peribronchial infiltration (**4.1**). Airway oedema and excess mucus production cause peripheral airways to become occluded, and atelectasis and collapse are not unusual findings (**4.2**).

Outcome

The natural history is an illness lasting about 10 days with cough persisting for a further 2–3 weeks. For those admitted to hospital, a small percentage will require intubation and ventilation for a median of 5 days. In developed countries, 30–60% of children develop recurrent viral wheezing following severe RSV infection.

Bordetella infection

Whooping cough is an acute respiratory infection characterized by paroxysmal episodes of coughing that may continue for many weeks. The vast majority of infections are caused by *Bordetella pertussis* but other *Bordetella* species, e.g. *B. parapertussis*, may produce a similar illness.

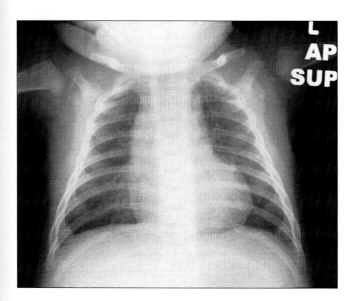

4.1 Respiratory syncytial virus bronchiolitis in a 6-month-old child. Chest X-ray shows chest hyperexpansion with peribronchial infiltration.

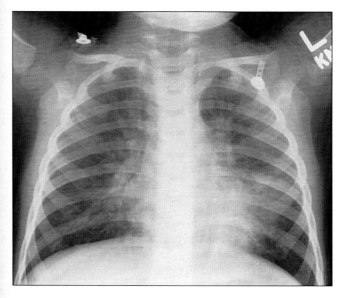

4.2 Severe respiratory syncytial virus lower respiratory infection in a 10-month-old child. Chest X-ray shows chest hyperexpansion, bronchial wall thickening and diffuse segmental atelectasis.

The illness is in three stages:

1. *The catarrhal stage*: low-grade fever, coryza, sneezing, mild cough, malaise and general flu-like symptoms. Erythromycin given at this stage may ameliorate symptoms and does eradicate nasopharyngeal carriage, thus reducing infectivity.
2. *The paroxysmal stage*: attacks of repetitive coughing during expiration, which may induce cyanosis, neck vein distension, lacrimation, drooling and post-tussive vomiting. Rapid inspiration through a partially closed glottis during inspiration causes the characteristic whoop after a coughing bout.
3. *The convalescent phase*: cough paroxysms may persist at a lower frequency and are frequently exacerbated by intercurrent illness.

Chest X-ray may be normal (in 25%) or demonstrate peribronchial consolidation, atelectasis and hilar lymphadenopathy.

Pneumonia

Incidence
Together, the available data for the developed world suggest an incidence of 10–15 cases/1000 children/year and a hospital admission rate of 1–4/1000 children/year. Both incidence and admission rates are greatest in the youngest children and rapidly fall after the age of 5 years.

Mortality
Death from pneumonia in previously well children is very rare in the developed world. In 1999 in England, 46 otherwise healthy children died from pneumonia (a death rate of 1.6/100 000 children/year). In the developing world, the incidence is 10 times higher and responsible for an estimated 5 million deaths annually in children under 5 years.

Severity assessment
Hypoxaemia in a child with pneumonia is a key indicator of severity with an increased mortality risk. An oxygen saturation of <92% in air, together with signs of severe disease or dehydration, are the cardinal indications for hospital admission. Increasing hypoxia, hypercarbia, exhaustion, apnoea or systemic shock are the principal

Table 4.1 BTS Guidelines for the Management of Community Acquired Pneumonia in Childhood

Severity assessment

Indications for admission to hospital in infants:
- oxygen saturation <92%, cyanosis;
- respiratory rate >70 breaths/min;
- difficulty in breathing;
- intermittent apnoea, grunting;
- not feeding;
- family not able to provide appropriate observation or supervision.

Indications for admission to hospital in older children:
- oxygen saturation <92%, cyanosis;
- respiratory rate >50 breaths/min;
- difficulty in breathing;
- grunting;
- signs of dehydration;
- family not able to provide appropriate observation or supervision.

Indications for transfer to intensive care facility:
- The patient is failing to maintain an SaO_2 of >92% in an FiO_2 of >0.6.
- The patient is shocked.
- There is a rising respiratory rate and rising pulse rate with clinical evidence of severe respiratory distress and exhaustion, with or without a raised arterial carbon dioxide tension ($PaCO_2$).
- There is recurrent apnoea or slow irregular breathing.

Thorax 2002; **57**: i1–i24

indications for transfer to an intensive care facility. British Thoracic Society (BTS) recommendations for admission to hospital and intensive care are shown in *Table 4.1*.

Aetiology

Pneumonias may be classified as viral, bacterial or atypical. Even the most recent and detailed aetiological studies fail to identify a causative organism in >20% of cases.

Viral pneumonia

Viruses are responsible for a large proportion of childhood pneumonias, particularly in children <2 years of age. In a UK study, viral aetiology was demonstrated in 71% of all pneumonias with a confirmed pathogen (37% of total).

RSV accounts for between 14% and 40% of all viral isolations and is an important pathogen in all pneumonia studies. Infants with severe RSV disease usually present with bronchiolitis. In a study of 140 cases of RSV lower respiratory infection, pneumonia defined as infiltration of the lung on chest X-ray was present in 54% of cases, suggesting infants with severe disease will often have a combination of bronchiolitis and interstitial pneumonia.

Parainfluenza 1, 2 and 3 together account for 15–20% of viral pneumonias, influenza A and B for between 8% and 27%, and adenovirus for 5–9% of viral pneumonias. Measles virus may cause a severe lower respiratory infection. The contribution of rhinovirus to lower respiratory infections is difficult to establish since it can often be isolated in asymptomatic children. Only 8% of hMPV-infected children with lower respiratory infection have evidence of pneumonia.

Clinical features

Viruses cause an interstitial pneumonia. Alveolar walls become thickened and sloughing of cells and infiltration of inflammatory cells occlude the alveoli. Decreased compliance and airway obstruction necessitate increased inspiratory pressures to maintain gas exchange, leading, in the presence of a compliant chest wall, to recession.

Viral pneumonia classically presents with respiratory distress, hyperexpansion, bilateral inspiratory crackles and expiratory wheeze. Hypoxia is common and may persist for several weeks.

Radiological features

There is hyperexpansion, interstitial infiltration with bronchial wall thickening and often focal areas of atelectasis or collapse (**4.3**). Chest X-rays are poor at discriminating between bacterial and viral pneumonia, up to half of children with interstitial infiltration on chest X-ray having evidence of bacterial pneumonia.

Outcome

Tachypnoea, irritant cough and wheeze may last for several weeks. However, the long-term prognosis, with the exception of disease caused by adenovirus (see later), is excellent.

Bacterial pneumonia

Aetiology

Bacteria are responsible for about 50% of pneumonias in hospitalized children. *Streptococcus pneumoniae* is the

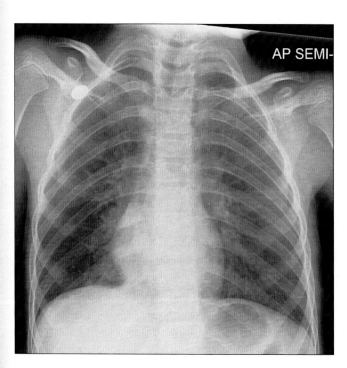

4.3 Viral pneumonia in an 8-year-old child. Chest X-ray shows chest hyperexpansion with diffuse peribronchial infiltration.

commonest cause (16–37% of all pneumonias). *Haemophilus influenzae* type B is rare in the HiB vaccinated population. *Staphylococcus aureus* causes acute severe pneumonia almost exclusively in the first year of life. Group A streptococcal pneumonia classically complicates chickenpox. Other rarer organisms include *Klebsiella pneumoniae*, legionella species and *Moraxella catarrhalis*.

Clinical features

Children may initially have no symptoms or signs localizing to the chest but high fever and tachypnoea appear to have the best positive predictive value. The classical signs are dullness to percussion, bronchial breathing and crackles. Bacterial pneumonias classically cause lobar or segmental consolidation. As this does not affect lung compliance or airway patency to the remaining healthy lung, signs of respiratory distress may be absent. Irritation of the pleural membranes or diaphragm may cause chest or abdominal pain. Wheezing is not a sign of primary bacterial pneumonia and suggests viral aetiology in younger children and possible atypical pneumonia in the older child.

Radiological features

Chest X-ray is effective at diagnosing bacterial pneumonia. It has a sensitivity of 75% and a specificity of between 40% and 100% in children admitted to hospital with clinical suspicion of pneumonia. However, defining aetiology on the basis of X-ray alone has been shown to be unreliable.

In lobar consolidation, the chest X-ray will show evidence of alveolar airspace disease and an air bronchogram, the result of a radiographically prominent interface between solid phase alveolar infiltrate and gas phase air-filled bronchioles.

Lung opacities may be localized to a particular lobe by the way they obscure neighbouring structures (**4.4–4.9**).

Atypical pneumonia

This is a term used principally to describe pneumonia caused by *Mycoplasma pneumoniae*. Other, rarer, organisms include *Chlamydia pneumoniae*, *Chlamydia psittacci*, *Legionella pneumophilia* and *Coxiella burnetti*.

Mycoplasma pneumoniae

Mycoplasma pneumonia accounts for between 9% and 42% of community acquired pneumonia in children. It is generally seen in epidemic years, which may explain the variation in incidence between studies. Infection typically affects children over the age of 5 years.

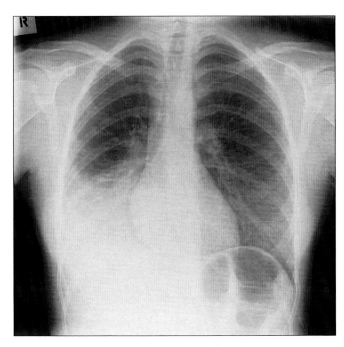

4.4 Right lower lobe pneumonia may obscure the right hemi-diaphragm and may be demarcated superiorly by the horizontal fissure. This chest X-ray shows dense consolidation of the right lower zone with obliteration of the right hemi-diaphragm and preservation of the right heart border (which is lost in middle lobe disease).

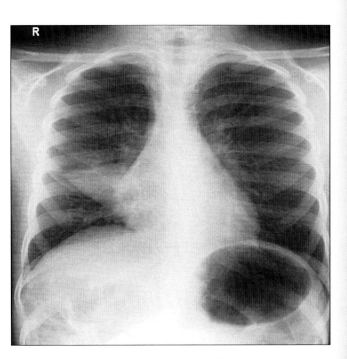

4.5 Right middle lobe pneumonia. Chest X-ray shows consolidation of the right mid zone with classical partial obliteration of the right heart border.

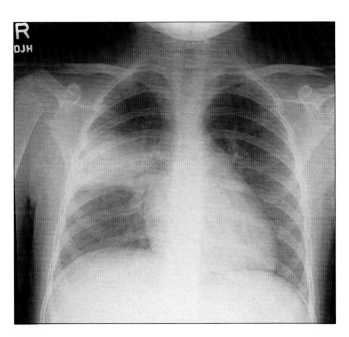

4.6 Right upper lobe pneumonia. Chest X-ray shows dense consolidation of the right mid zone delineated inferiorly by the horizontal fissure. There is sparing of the apical segment of the right upper lobe.

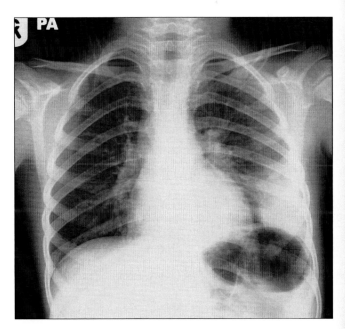

4.7 Left lower lobe pneumonia. Chest X-ray shows dense peripheral consolidation in the left lower zone with obliteration of the left hemi-diaphragm and preservation of the left heart border. In some cases, consolidation may only be visible behind the heart.

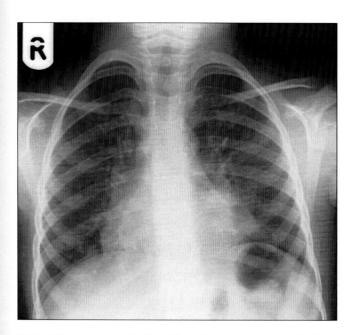

4.8 Left lingular consolidation. Chest X-ray shows consolidation in the left mid zone with partial obliteration of the left heart border.

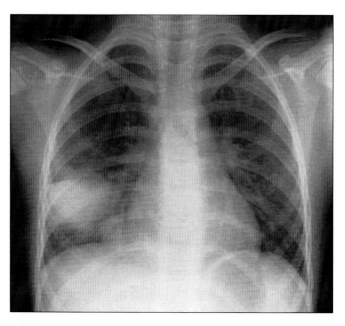

4.9 Round pneumonia, commonly caused by pneumococcus. Chest X-ray shows well demarcated round peripheral consolidation in the right mid zone. These pneumonias may be more difficult to localize to a specific lobe.

Chlamydia pneumoniae

C. pneumoniae is increasingly recognized as an important pathogen in both children and adults, and has recently been shown to be responsible for 9–20% of all cases of pneumonia in children.

Clinical features

Up to 20% of infections caused by mycoplasma are asymptomatic. However, both mycoplasma and chlamydia infections commonly present with pharyngitis and laryngitis. Pneumonia causes a largely non-productive cough, fever and crackles and may cause wheezing and retrosternal pain. Average duration of illness is about 2 weeks although the cough may persist for over a month. Mycoplasma has many potential extrapulmonary manifestations, including myocarditis, pericarditis, erythema multiforme, haemolytic anaemia, arthritis, glomerulonephritis and central nervous system disease.

Radiological features

X-ray findings are highly variable. Classically, atypical pneumonias cause a symmetrical reticulonodular infiltrate on chest X-ray representing interstitial bronchopneumonia

(**4.10**). However, lobar consolidation and hilar lymphadenopathy have also been described. Pleural effusion is rare (<15%).

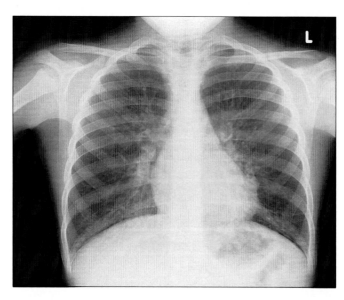

4.10 Mycoplasma pneumonia. Chest X-ray shows symmetrical reticulonodular infiltrates consistent with interstitial pneumonia.

Mixed bacterial and viral infection

Mixed infections either of bacterium and virus, or of two different viruses or bacteria, account for between 10% and 40% of pneumonia cases in children, and coinfection probably has an important influence on disease severity. Influenza, in particular, is classically associated with *S. aureus* superinfection, and possibly also in severe cases of pneumococcal pneumonia.

Investigation

A chest X-ray is not necessary for children who have mild acute lower respiratory tract infection not requiring admission to hospital.

Children requiring hospital admission for pneumonia should have the following investigations:

- pulse oximetry
- chest X-ray
- blood cultures
- viral antigen detection and viral polymerase chain reaction from nasopharyngeal aspirate – in all children under 18 months of age (highly specific)
- urea and electrolytes: in patients who are severely ill, hyponatraemia is common and may indicate inappropriate antidiuretic hormone secretion and necessitate fluid restriction.

Determining the causative organism in community acquired pneumonia is not straightforward in children:

- yield is low (<10%) from blood cultures
- sputum samples are often inadequate and may be confounded by upper respiratory tract colonization
- serological responses are poor in patients under 1 year of age
- urinary and plasma antigen detection tests are unreliable.

Acute phase reactants are commonly measured but great variation exists in the acute phase response to both bacterial and viral infection making sensitivity and specificity of tests poor.

Management

Management is largely supportive. British Thoracic Society guidelines are outlined in *Table 4.2*.

Acute complications of lower respiratory infection

If a child remains febrile after 48 hours of treatment for pneumonia, reassessment is necessary.

The potential causes of persistent illness include:

- *Treatment failure.* The child may be receiving inadequate antibiotic treatment. Although there have been recent concerns regarding penicillin-resistant strains of *S. pneumoniae*, standard IV treatment achieves a serum concentration much greater than the minimum inhibiting concentration of most penicillin-resistant strains.
- *Development of complications.* Local complications include parapneumonic effusion and empyema, lung abscess and necrotizing pneumonia. Metastatic infection causing septicaemia, osteomyelitis and septic arthritis occurs rarely but should be considered particularly in *S. aureus* infection.
- *Predisposition to severe disease.* Rarely, failure to respond to appropriate treatment may reflect an underlying disorder such as cystic fibrosis or an immunodeficiency.

Parapneumonic effusion and empyema

Parapneumonic effusions develop in 40% of children who are admitted to hospital with bacterial pneumonia.

Clinical features

Children will have a persistent high fever and often chest/abdominal pain due to pleural/diaphragmatic irritation. Positional scoliosis, to guard the affected hemithorax, is common. Large parapneumonic collections may cause contralateral mediastinal shift. Classically there is ipsilateral dullness to percussion and reduced breath sounds on auscultation.

Radiological features

Obliteration of the costophrenic angle on erect chest X-ray is often the first sign of a pleural collection. With larger effusions, the underlying lung is obliterated by uniform opacity. Often the effusion is most evident as an accentuated pleural reflection seen laterally (**4.11A**). In younger children, anteroposterior chest X-rays are often taken in the supine position, in which case pleural fluid may cause little more than subtle uniform opacity across the hemithorax.

Table 4.2 BTS Guidelines for the Management of Community Acquired Pneumonia in Childhood

Management of lower respiratory infection in children

- The child cared for at home should be reviewed by a general practitioner if deteriorating or if not improving after 48 hours on treatment.
- Families of children who are well enough to be cared for at home need information on managing pyrexia, preventing dehydration and identifying any deterioration.
- Patients whose oxygen saturation is 92% or less while breathing air should be treated with oxygen given by nasal cannulae, head box or face mask to maintain oxygen saturation above 92%.
- Agitation may be an indication that the child is hypoxic.
- Nasogastric tubes may compromise breathing and should therefore be avoided in severely ill children and especially in infants with small nasal passages. If used, the smallest tube should be passed down the smallest nostril.
- Intravenous fluids, if needed, should be given at 80% basal levels and serum electrolytes monitored.
- Chest physiotherapy is not beneficial and should not be performed in children with pneumonia.
- Antipyretics and analgesics can be used to keep the child comfortable and to help coughing.
- In the ill child, minimal handling may reduce metabolic and oxygen requirements.
- Patients on oxygen therapy should have at least 4-hourly observations including oxygen saturation.

Antibiotic management

- Young children presenting with mild symptoms of lower respiratory tract infection need not be treated with antibiotics.
- Amoxicillin is first choice for oral antibiotic therapy in children under the age of 5 years because it is effective against the majority of pathogens which cause community acquired pneumonia (CAP) in this group, is well tolerated, and cheap. Alternatives are co-amoxiclav, cefaclor, erythromycin, clarithromycin and azithromycin.
- Because mycoplasma pneumonia is more prevalent in older children, macrolide antibiotics may be used as first-line empirical treatment in children aged 5 and above.
- Macrolide antibiotics should be used if either mycoplasma or chlamydia pneumonia is suspected.
- Amoxicillin should be used as first-line treatment at any age if *S. pneumoniae* is thought to be the likely pathogen.
- If *Staphylococcus aureus* is thought to be the likely pathogen, a macrolide or combination of flucloxacillin with amoxicillin is appropriate.
- Although there appears to be no difference in response to conventional antibiotic treatment in children with penicillin-resistant *S. pneumoniae*, the data are limited and the majority of children in these studies were not treated with oral β-lactam agents alone.
- Antibiotics administered orally are safe and effective for children presenting with CAP.
- Intravenous antibiotics should be used in the treatment of pneumonia in children when the child is unable to absorb oral antibiotics (for example, because of vomiting) or presents with severe signs and symptoms.
- Appropriate intravenous antibiotics for severe pneumonia include co-amoxiclav, cefuroxime and cefotaxime. If clinical or microbiological data suggest that *S. pneumoniae* is the causative organism, amoxicillin, ampicillin or penicillin alone may be used.
- In a patient who is receiving intravenous antibiotic therapy for the treatment of CAP, oral treatment should be considered if there is clear evidence of improvement.

From *Thorax* 2002; **57**: i1–i24, with permission

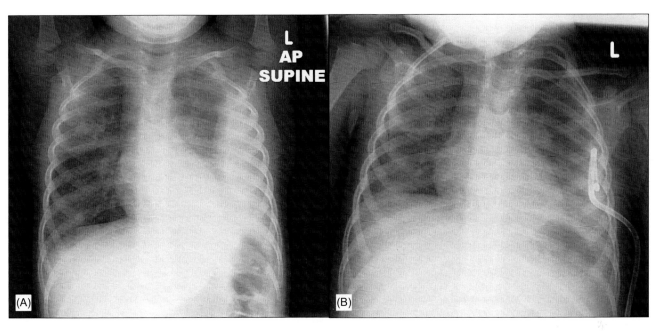

4.11 Left-sided pneumonia with empyema before (A) and after (B) pigtail drain insertion.

Effusions may be mobile or restricted in position. Dependent fluid visible on chest X-ray may represent a sterile parapneumonic effusion or empyema. Non-dependent fluid that does not change its configuration on erect positioning is likely to be a loculated non-mobile organizing empyema.

Ultrasonography is very useful in defining the properties of pleural fluid. It is capable of discriminating between pleural thickening and pleural fluid and can therefore accurately determine the amount of drainable fluid and the optimum position for drain insertion.

A computed tomography scan is not helpful in the routine management of parapneumonic effusion or empyema.

Management

Effusions that are enlarging or compromising respiratory function should be managed with drainage of the pleural space. Recent BTS guidelines suggest loculated parapneumonic effusion or empyema should be drained either by video-assisted thoracoscopy or by insertion of a pigtail catheter with administration of intrapleural urokinase (**4.11B, 4.12**). Both have a high success rate and a recent randomized controlled trial showed no difference in efficacy but fibrinolysis was less expensive.

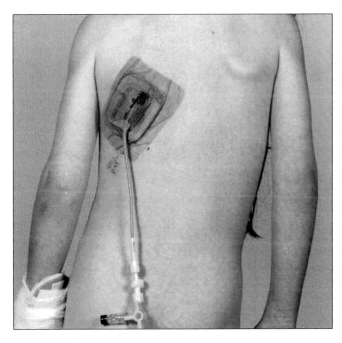

4.12 Pigtail chest drain *in situ* in a 4-year-old girl with left-sided empyema.

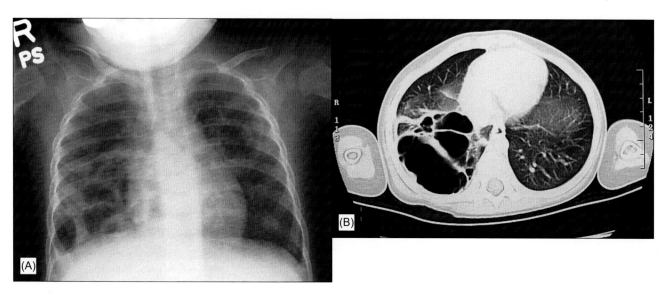

4.13 Chest X-ray (A) and high-resolution computed tomography (B) showing multiple pneumatocoeles post-staphylococcal pneumonia (most evident in the right lower zone and left middle zone).

Pneumatocoeles

Staphylococcus aureus presents with severe illness, and parapneumonic complications in up to 90% of cases. Destruction of bronchial walls and consequent air trapping may lead to pneumatocoele formation in up to 50% of cases. X-ray shows multiple radiolucent cavitations of the lung (**4.13A**), clearly evident on high-resolution computed tomography (**4.13B**). The prognosis is good, with complete resolution and normal lung function after a few months.

Lung abscess

Lung abscess is a rare complication of community acquired pneumonia and is usually caused by *S. aureus*. Viridans group streptococci, group A streptococcus and rarely *S. pneumoniae* have also been implicated. Mixed anaerobic bacteria are common in lung abscess associated with aspiration pneumonia.

X-ray shows a well-demarcated walled cavity with an air-fluid level (**4.14**). Prolonged intravenous antibiotic therapy usually settles the infection without further intervention. Cysts may be present in an otherwise well child for months. An important differential diagnosis of primary lung abscess is infection in a previously undiagnosed congenital cyst.

Chronic complications of lower respiratory infection

Bronchiolitis obliterans

This is the term ascribed to the chronic obstructive condition that may follow severe bronchiolitis and pneumonia. It is most commonly seen following lower respiratory infection with adenovirus, although it may also be caused by influenza virus and *Mycoplasma pneumoniae*. Histology reveals destruction of muscle and elastic tissue, and fibrosis of the bronchiole wall. The terminal bronchioles are obstructed by fibrous tissue and the distal respiratory bronchioles consequently become dilated. There is patchy overdistention, atelectasis and collapse at the alveolar level. Symptoms and signs persist for months with wheezing, chest exacerbations and localized signs on auscultation (**4.15**).

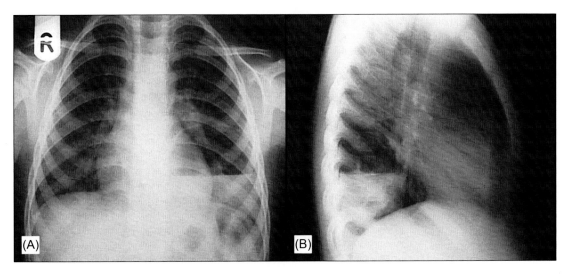

4.14 Anteroposterior (A) and lateral (B) chest X-rays showing a large lung abscess with air–fluid level, in the left lower lobe. Abscesses are generally thick-walled structures.

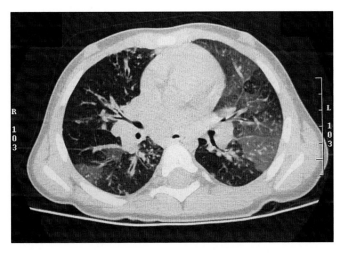

4.15 Bronchiolitis obliterans post-adenoviral pneumonia in a 6-year-old girl. High-resolution computed tomography scans show bronchial wall thickening, bronchial dilatation and mosaicism suggestive of air trapping and redistribution of pulmonary blood flow.

Bronchiectasis

Bronchiectasis is characterized by bronchial dilatation accompanied by a chronic productive cough. It may be the result of countless different insults to the lung, but it is well described as a long-term complication of pneumonia requiring hospitalization. Children hospitalized for pneumonia are 15 times more likely to develop bronchiectasis in the future. Bronchiectasis is described in more detail elsewhere (see Chapters 6 and 7).

Further reading

Balfour-Lynn IM, Abrahamson E, Cohen G, *et al*. BTS guidelines for the management of pleural infection in children. *Thorax* 2005; 60(Suppl 1): i1–21.

British Thoracic Society Guidelines for the Management of Community Acquired Pneumonia in Childhood. *Thorax* 2002; 57(Suppl 1): i1–24.

McIntosh K. Community-acquired pneumonia in children. *N Engl J Med* 2002; 346: 429–37.

Sinaniotis CA, Sinaniotis AC. Community-acquired pneumonia in children. *Curr Opin Pulm Med* 2005; 11: 218–25.

Sonnappa S, Cohen G, Owens CM, *et al*. Comparison of urokinase and video-assisted thoracoscopic surgery for treatment of childhood empyema. *Am J Respir Crit Care Med* 2006; 174: 221–7.

Williams JV, Harris PA, Tollefson SJ, *et al*. Human metapneumovirus and lower respiratory tract disease in otherwise healthy infants and children. *N Engl J Med* 2004; 350: 443–50.

Chapter 5

Tuberculosis

Siobhán B. Carr

Introduction

Mycobacterium tuberculosis (TB) is a worldwide problem with a long history, which still causes high rates of morbidity and mortality; an estimated 1.6 million people die each year from this potentially curable disease (World Health Organization [WHO]: www.who.int/tb/en). Early treatment consisted of rest (often in a TB sanatorium), sun and fresh air. In the early twentieth century, surgical collapse of the affected lung, with the aim of creating an anaerobic environment to kill the organism was commonplace. Streptomycin was one of the first antibiotics to be discovered in the 1940s and was quickly applied as the treatment of TB; it continues to play an occasional role in treatment to the present day.

Extent of the problem

The incidence of *Mycobacterium tuberculosis* varies across the globe, although it is generally more common in poorer socioeconomic groups. The incidence and mortality of new cases in developing countries is much higher than in Western society (*Table 5.1*). Figure **5.1** shows the WHO figures for new and relapse cases of TB in 2005. Countries with a high incidence, particularly sub-Saharan Africa, have the added burden of a high prevalence of HIV; an individual with HIV is 50 times more likely to develop TB than one without. Globally, the prevalence of HIV infection in individuals with TB is about 11%.

Another emerging problem worldwide is the development of drug-resistant forms of TB. Multidrug-resistant TB (MDR TB) refers to strains that are resistant to at least rifampicin and isoniazid, two of the first-line drugs in TB treatment. Twenty per cent of worldwide samples from 2000 to 2004 were found to be MDR. Two per cent were extremely drug-resistant strains (XDR TB; an MDR strain with added resistance to quinolones and at least one of the injectable second-line therapies, e.g. amikacin (WHO 2007 data)).

Aetiology and spread

Childhood TB usually represents a recent infection. Spread is by inhalation of the bacterium, commonly from an infected adult within the family; the closer the contact and the longer the exposure, the more likely the infection.

Table 5.1 World Health Organization reported incidence and mortality from *Mycobacterium tuberculosis* in 2005		
Region	Incidence per 100 000 population	Mortality per 100 000 population
Africa	343	74
South-east Asia	181	31
Western Pacific	110	17
Eastern Mediterranean	104	21
Europe	50	7.4
Americas	39	5.5
Global	136	24

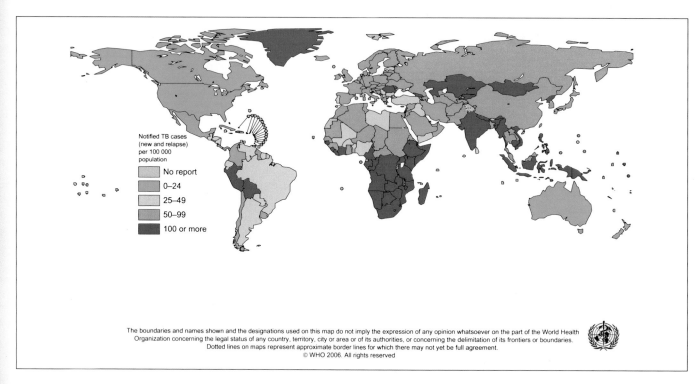

5.1 Map of tuberculosis notification rates for new and relapse cases in 2005 (courtesy of WHO, 2006: www.who.int/tb/en).

In the majority, the organism induces immunity rather than disease; asymptomatic individuals are considered to have latent TB, estimated to be present in one-third of the world population. Alternatively, inhalation can lead to a delayed hypersensitivity reaction in the peripheral lung, which forms a localized granuloma, consisting of epithelioid cells and activated T cells. Enlargement of a regional lymph node in this initial reaction is known as the primary complex (**5.2**). In the majority of children this resolves spontaneously; some calcification is often apparent (the Gohn focus). A small number caseate, which may lead either to localized pulmonary, pleural or pericardial infection, or to haematogenous spread to bone, central nervous system or other areas of pulmonary tissue (miliary TB).

Post-primary TB is a reactivation, usually several years after the primary infection and is most commonly pulmonary. Poor nutrition or poor health, particularly in those with lowered immunity, e.g. HIV-infected individuals, are predisposing factors. About 10% of individuals with latent TB will develop TB disease during their lifetime; this is the typical clinical picture in adults who will often have cavitating lung disease, and is also seen in some older children. At this stage, the infection is most likely to be transmissible.

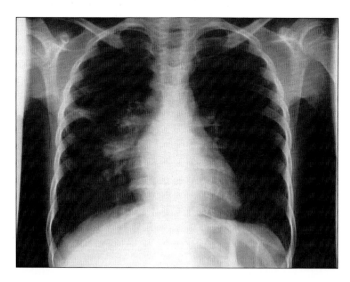

5.2 Chest X-ray of a 6-year-old child showing primary complex (peripheral shadowing and enlarged hilar lymph node).

Presentation

Common systemic symptoms and signs include weight loss, fatigue, anorexia, night sweats and fevers (which may be low grade). HIV infection may mask the presentation. TB must always be borne in mind in children with HIV and the converse also applies.

Pulmonary

Two-thirds of paediatric TB notifications in England and Wales are for pulmonary disease. Symptoms localized to the chest include persistent cough (common), chest pain or haemoptysis (less common particularly in younger children). Onset of signs and symptoms over weeks to months is characteristic. Occasionally, localized compression of an airway with distal infection can lead to an acute pneumonia-like presentation. Infections that fail to respond to conventional treatment or occur in children from high-risk ethnic groups should arouse suspicion of TB. Hilar lymphadenopathy or erythema nodosum (**5.3**) are classical clues to the diagnosis. The latter is a raised, painful, cutaneous lesion, which is caused by inflammation of the fatty layer of the skin, usually on the shins and may be a delayed hypersensitivity reaction. Miliary tuberculosis (**5.4**) is most common in the younger child. Chest symptoms may be absent, although the child is often sick, febrile and hypoxic.

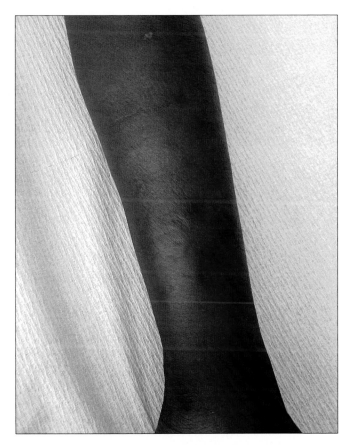

5.3 Erythema nodosum on the shins of an 8-year-old child who first presented with these painful raised erythematous lumps on both shins. There were no respiratory symptoms but on questioning there had been some weight loss and tiredness. Mantoux test was strongly positive with induration of 22 mm and chest X-ray showed unilateral hilar adenopathy.

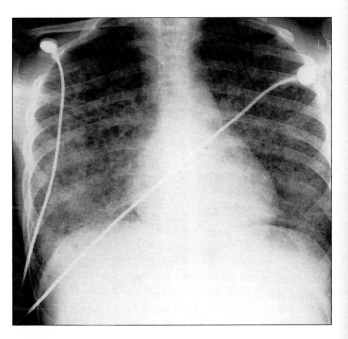

5.4 Chest X-ray of miliary tuberculosis in a teenager, who required ventilatory support. A Mantoux test had been negative 3 weeks before presentation. This was performed as contact tracing. The sibling had presented 1 month before with pulmonary tuberculosis; they had shared a bedroom and demonstrate that tuberculosis can occasionally be acquired from child-to-child spread.

Extrapulmonary

Mycobacterium tuberculosis can present as a slowly swelling, painless lymph node or mass of nodes (**5.5**), commonly in the neck, with or without systemic signs and symptoms. Bony involvement is often of the spine (**5.6**), which may lead to local or referred pain; for example, spinal TB with involvement of the surrounding tissue and psoas muscle (cold abscess) can lead to presentation with a limp. Children with central nervous system involvement may present with decreased levels of consciousness and signs of raised intercranial pressure. Tuberculous meningitis should be suspected in children with indolent prodromes prior to an acute presentation. All cases of non-pulmonary TB require a chest X-ray because pulmonary involvement is a common association.

Investigation

Clinical suspicion is key; the diagnosis is most commonly delayed because it has not been considered. Confirmation of the diagnosis is carried out using a variety of methods:

- tuberculin skin testing
- radiological imaging
- microbiological testing
- histological analysis
- immunological blood tests.

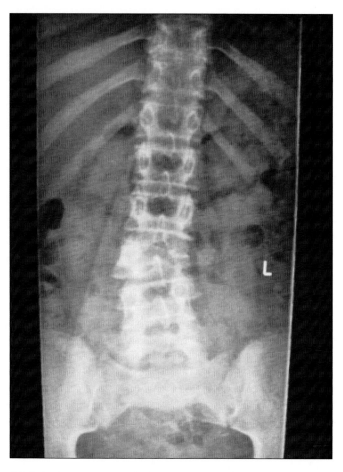

5.6 Spinal tuberculosis of the third lumbar vertebra, demonstrating collapse of the body of the vertebra. This 9-year-old child had an 8-month history of back pain prior to biopsy diagnosis of tuberculosis.

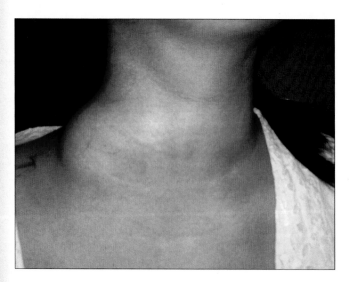

5.5 Swollen tuberculosis lymph nodes in the neck of a teenager with night sweats and weight loss over the preceding month.

Non-specific markers of infection and inflammation, e.g. C-reactive protein and erythrocyte sedimentation rate may be raised, but lack sensitivity and specificity.

Tuberculin skin testing

The Mantoux tuberculin skin test is based on a delayed hypersensitivity reaction to purified protein derivative of tuberculin. A standard volume and strength of purified protein derivative is injected intradermally. Sensitized subjects will develop an erythema and induration; the latter should be measured between 48 and 72 hours later across the arm (**5.7**). In children, >6 mm is considered a positive test, unless they have received BCG vaccination when the cut-off is 15 mm (National Institute for Health and Clinical Excellence [NICE] Guidance: www.nice.org.uk/CG033). A strongly positive tuberculin skin test can result in blistering

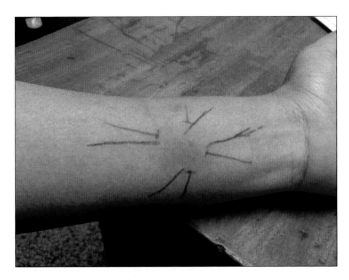

5.7 Positive tuberculin skin test (Mantoux) – usually placed on the left forearm. The measurement is taken across the indurated area (measure between marks made by drawing on the skin in a line until the induration is hit), not the red area.

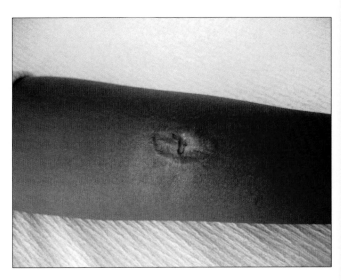

5.8 Localized scarring following strongly positive tuberculin skin test.

and scarring (**5.8**); after measuring, this can be treated with a mild steroid cream. The test may be negative in over 10% of patients with active TB, particularly those with HIV, severe malnutrition or taking systemic corticosteroids.

Imaging

Pulmonary TB is diagnosed in the presence of abnormal chest X-ray or computed tomography findings. However, findings are highly variable and may mimic pneumonia or empyema (**5.9**). Hilar lymphadenopathy (**5.10**) is a common finding although may be more clearly visualized on computed tomography than plain radiograph. Magnetic resonance imaging is most commonly employed for spinal imaging (**5.11**) and ultrasound can be useful for imaging suspect lymph nodes. Computed tomography guided biopsy may be useful for paraspinal collections.

Microbiology

The importance of a microbiological diagnosis can not be overemphasized. The incidence of multidrug or single drug resistance is increasing and appropriate identification of *Mycobacterium tuberculosis* and its sensitivities is a priority.

A microbiological diagnosis should therefore be sought in all cases. Although in children the likelihood of having smear-positive TB is low, cavitating lung disease is seen in older children and teenagers. Attempts to collect three

consecutive sputum samples should be made; nebulized hypertonic saline can aid expectoration in younger children. Alternatively, early morning gastric aspirates via nasogastric tube on three consecutive days can be performed, and

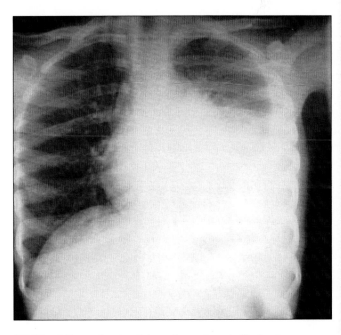

5.9 Chest X-ray showing tuberculous pleural effusion in a 7-year-old child.

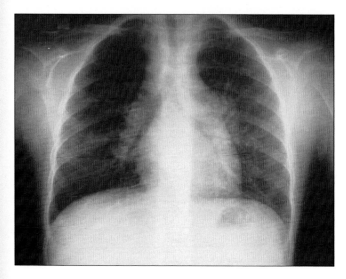

5.10 Chest X-ray showing bilateral hilar lymphadenopathy.

bronchoalveolar lavage should be considered. With these collection techniques, between 25% and 50% of infected children have mycobacterium identified.

Histopathology samples (from lymph nodes or biopsies) may show mycobacterium or necrotic or caseating granulomatous material highly suggestive of TB. In lymph node infection caused by *Mycobacterium tuberculosis*, full anti-TB treatment will still be necessary even if the whole node is removed. Pleural fluid or occasionally ascitic fluid, when present, should be obtained for culture or polymerase chain reaction.

Acid-fast bacilli are identified using a fluorescent auramine (**5.12**) or Ziehl–Neelsen stain (**5.13**) of sputum, gastric aspirates or biopsies. Rapid (2-week) liquid culture techniques are now available, replacing or running in parallel with the much slower Lowenstein–Jensen medium, which can take up to 8 weeks to grow the organisms. Rapid diagnostic techniques can also give early identification of rifampicin-resistant strains; the majority of these will be MDR strains.

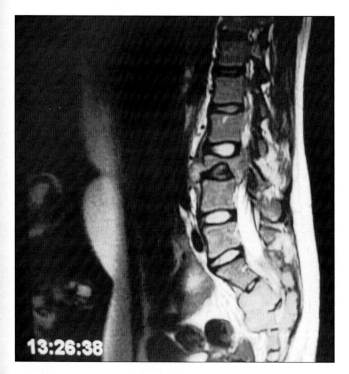

5.11 Spinal magnetic resonance imaging of the child whose spinal X-ray is shown in **5.6**. T2-weighted image showing relative sparing of the discs but collapse of both L3 and several sacral vertebrae. Dual site tuberculosis of the spine is unusual.

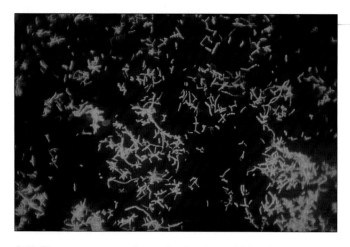

5.12 Fluorescent auramine stain showing acid-fast bacilli.

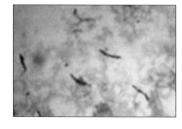

5.13 Ziehl–Neelsen-stained sample obtained from a gastric aspirate from a child.

Polymerase chain reaction

Polymerase chain reaction may be used as an adjunct in the diagnosis of TB; it has good specificity but a low sensitivity of about 75%. It may be most useful when searching for TB in fluid collected from non-airway samples such as cerebrospinal fluid, pleural effusions or ascites.

Immunological tests: gamma interferon tests

Recently, novel blood-based diagnostic tests have been developed. These tests measure gamma interferon production from stimulated peripheral blood T cells; there is some concern that diagnostic accuracy may be lower in individuals infected with HIV. The antigens detected are specific for *Mycobacterium tuberculosis* and are not found in BCG-inoculated, non-infected patients. Their use is becoming more widespread in the developed world and they are now included in NICE guidelines, although work on their accuracy and exact use in tuberculous disease, rather than latent TB, continues.

Prevention and contact tracing

In many areas of the world, there are active BCG immunization programmes. This strategy appears to be most useful in preventing miliary and central nervous system infection. Localized reactions to neonatal immunization with BCG are common; they will often discharge several times over several months. No treatment is necessary apart from reassurance and watchful waiting, while the lesion slowly resolves.

Contact tracing is organized for all close contacts of adults or children with active disease. Close family members and contacts of infected children should be traced, not because the child is likely to be infectious but because they are most likely to have acquired the disease from an infected adult contact.

Treatment

Guidelines for treatment are available in most countries although the basic principle has remained the same for some years. In the UK, the National Institute for Health and Clinical Excellence has recently published recommendations. A 6-month treatment regimen is used for most cases comprising 2 months of quadruple

therapy (isoniazid, rifampicin, ethambutol, pyrazinamide), followed by 4 months of dual therapy with isoniazid and rifampicin. Culture results are usually back by 2 months and the remaining period of treatment can be tailored to suit sensitivity patterns. Up to 2 years of tailored therapy is used in patients with MDR TB (**5.14**). Extended courses of a year are used for central nervous system involvement and occasionally bony TB. Directly observed therapy using a three times per week regimen of standard drugs, a strategy favoured by the World Health Organization, may be used in children who are poorly compliant.

Chemoprophylaxis

Chemoprophylaxis is used in latent TB, which is usually found during contact tracing or on new immigrant screening. These children have a positive tuberculin skin test but no evidence of disease; gamma interferon tests are used to confirm this. Chemoprophylaxis comprises either 3 months of isoniazid and rifampicin or 6 months of isoniazid alone.

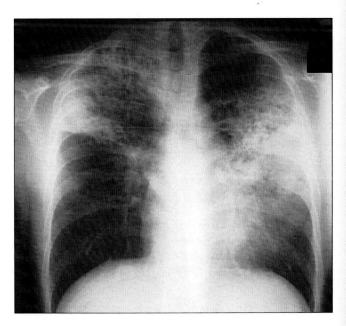

5.14 Chest X-ray showing extensive pulmonary involvement in a 15-year-old with multidrug-resistant tuberculosis.

Chapter 6

Cystic fibrosis

Jane C. Davies

Introduction

Cystic fibrosis (CF) affects 7000 people in the UK and about 30 000 in the USA, making it the commonest autosomal recessive disease of Caucasians. Presentation and clinical course is variable, ranging from classic, severe, multi-organ disease through to milder and single organ manifestations. Conventional management has advanced to improve the prognosis for patients significantly in recent decades, although the disease still carries a significant treatment burden.

The basic defect

The cystic fibrosis gene

The gene responsible for CF is located on chromosome 7q31.2 and was cloned in 1989 and named CF transmembrane conductance regulator (*CFTR*). More than 1200 disease-causing mutations have been detected in the *CFTR* gene, which can be divided into five classes (**6.1**). The major mutation, present in approximately 70% of CF chromosomes worldwide, is a deletion of phenylalanine at position 508 (ΔF508, more recently termed Phe508del), although its frequency varies greatly among different ethnic groups.

The cystic fibrosis transmembrane conductance regulator protein and disease pathophysiology

CFTR is expressed in the apical membrane of epithelial cells, including airway and intestinal epithelium, where it functions as a cyclic adenosine monophosphate-regulated chloride channel (**6.2**). In addition, CFTR has a number of other functions, some of them incompletely understood, including regulation of other ion channels such as the epithelial sodium channel (ENaC) and calcium-activated chloride channels (CaCC) (*Table 6.1*). Loss of inhibition of ENaC leads to hyperabsorption of sodium (and thus water down its osmotic gradient), which, together with impaired chloride ion secretion, results in dehydration of the airway surface liquid, the so-called low volume hypothesis (**6.3**) of pathophysiology.

Making the diagnosis

Sweat testing

Sweat Na^+ and Cl^- are raised in CF due to a failure of CFTR in the sweat gland to absorb chloride. This observation has led to the development of the sweat test as the gold standard for diagnosis (*Table 6.2*). Methods include the classical pilocarpine iontopheresis of Gibson and Cooke, and more recently the Macroduct collection system (**6.4**);

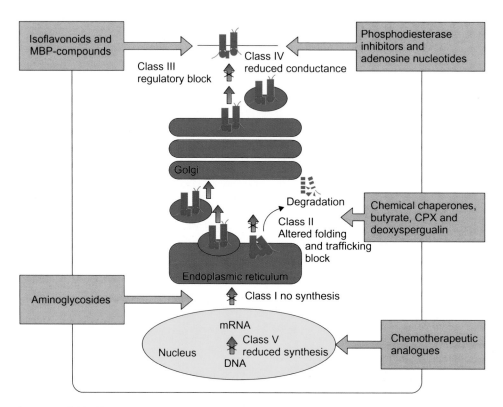

6.1 *CFTR* gene mutations are divided into classes depending on the effect on protein production; for many of these, novel therapeutic strategies are being explored. Class I (premature stop mutations) lead to no full length protein; certain drugs, including members of the aminoglycoside group of antibiotics and the new orally active agent, PTC124, have been shown to over-ride the 'stop' instruction and lead to partial restoration of protein function. Class II mutations lead to misfolded protein, which is degraded and fails to reach the apical membrane of the cell. ΔF508 is the commonest example of this class worldwide; so-called 'chemical chaperones' can allow the abnormal CFTR to traffic to the cell surface where it is partially functional. Classes III and IV lead to protein at the cell surface, which functions suboptimally, and Class V mutations (not shown) lead to low levels of protein being produced. Classes IV and V are more commonly associated with a degree of *CFTR* function and patients are often pancreatic sufficient. Reproduced with permission from Choo-Kang LR, Zeitlin PL. Type I, II, III, IV and V cystic fibrosis transmembrane conductance regulator defects and opportunities for therapy. *Curr Opin Pulm Med* 2000; 6: 521–9.

Table 6.1 Recognized functions of CFTR

Function	Proposed association with disease
Chloride ion transport	Reduced ASL height; impaired MCC
Regulation of	
ENaC/ORCC/CaCC	Reduced ASL height; impaired MCC
Adenosine triphosphate release	Disrupted paracrine signalling
Bicarbonate transport	Increased acidity of airway secretions
Transport of glutathione	Redox imbalance
Role in sulphation/sialylation processes	Increased mucus viscosity
	Increased abundance of asialoGM1 receptors (bacterial adherence or inflammatory signalling)
Role in lung development?	Unclear

ASL, airway surface liquid; MCC, mucociliary clearance.

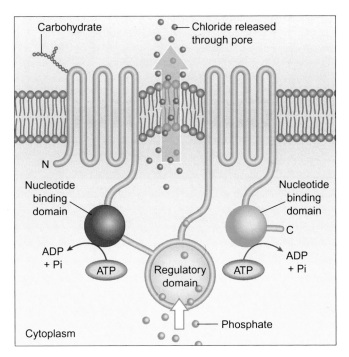

6.2 Pictorial representation of cystic fibrosis transmembrane conductance regulator structure.

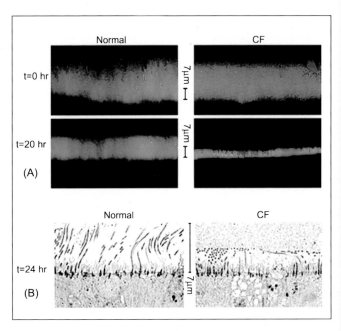

6.3 The low-volume hypothesis of cystic fibrosis disease pathogenesis. A fixed volume of liquid (green) applied to the apical surface of cultured cells is significantly reduced above cystic fibrosis cells after 20–24 hours (A). Potentially proinflammatory stimuli (red) such as bacteria are able to interact directly with the cell surface and ciliary function is impaired as cilia are no longer able to fully extend (B) (modified with permission from Matsui H, Grubb BR, Tarran R, *et al.* Evidence for periciliary liquid layer depletion, not abnormal ion composition, in the pathogenesis of cystic fibrosis airways disease. *Cell* 1998; 95: 1005–15).

such newer techniques require much smaller volumes of sweat, particularly in small children. Tests should be performed in duplicate; an unequivocally abnormal result is sweat chloride >60 mmol; normal values are <40 mmol, although some groups advocate reducing the normal cut-off to 30 mmol, particularly in infants. Depending on the degree of clinical suspicion, other supportive tests may be required.

Cystic fibrosis transmembrane conductance regulator genotype

DNA analysis can confirm the diagnosis (two disease-causing mutations) but cannot exclude it unless the whole of the *CFTR* gene is sequenced, which is largely impractical outside the context of research studies. Although certain mutations can be classified as 'mild' on the basis of epidemiological studies, individual prognostication is to be

Table 6.2 Conditions that are characterized by elevated sweat electrolyte concentrations. In practice, the two most common causes of a false positive test are eczema and artefact. In most cases, confusion with cystic fibrosis is very unlikely

- Cystic fibrosis
- Eczema
- Untreated adrenal insufficiency
- Type 1 glycogen storage disease
- Nephrogenic diabetes insipidus
- Malnutrition
- Panhypopituitarism
- Acquired immunodeficiency syndrome
- Artefact (incorrectly performed sweat test)
- Fucoscidosis
- Hypothyroidism
- Ectodermal dysplasia
- Mucopolysaccharidosis

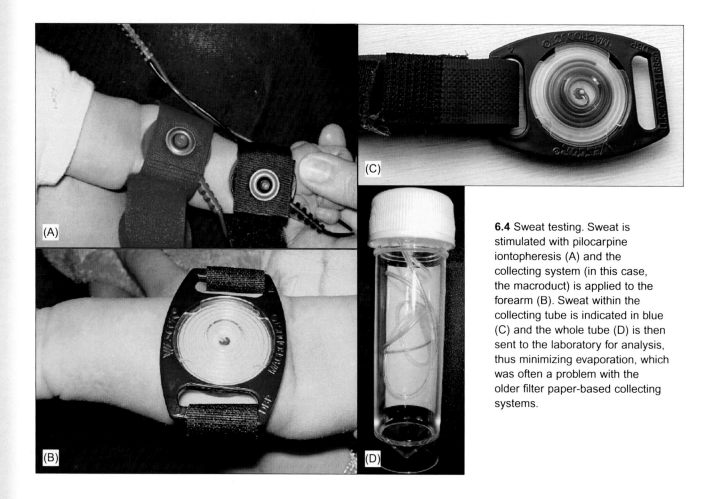

6.4 Sweat testing. Sweat is stimulated with pilocarpine iontopheresis (A) and the collecting system (in this case, the macroduct) is applied to the forearm (B). Sweat within the collecting tube is indicated in blue (C) and the whole tube (D) is then sent to the laboratory for analysis, thus minimizing evaporation, which was often a problem with the older filter paper-based collecting systems.

avoided as, in particular, the respiratory phenotype can be variable with all mutations.

Stool elastase

In a patient presenting with failure to thrive, a normal stool elastase makes the diagnosis of CF unlikely as this test is abnormally low in pancreatic sufficient CF. It is also useful once the diagnosis has been established to confirm the pancreatic status of a patient.

Nasal potential difference measurements

The abnormal potential difference (PD) across mucosal surfaces can be measured by passing a soft catheter under the inferior turbinate. Normal values for baseline readings are 0 to –30 mV whereas CF readings are higher (more negative) than –34 mV. The diagnosis can be further refined by perfusing the nose with solutions of amiloride to block sodium transport, and isoprenaline/low chloride to stimulate CFTR (**6.5**). Nasal potential difference

measurements require extensive experience if results are to be accurate and they are often uninterpretable if the patient has an upper respiratory tract infection, chronic rhinitis or nasal polyps.

Neonatal screening

The evidence for the value of neonatal screening for the disease has come from a number of retrospective trials, all showing benefit, but with the disadvantage of using historical controls. There has been one prospective, randomized trial from Wisconsin, USA in which 650 341 babies were screened. Of 96 infants in whom a diagnosis of CF was made, in 56 the diagnosis was communicated to the parents at once, and in 40 the diagnosis was suppressed, allowing it to be made on clinical grounds. There were small but clear-cut nutritional benefits in the group in which the screening diagnosis was communicated, persisting to 10 years of age. The benefits

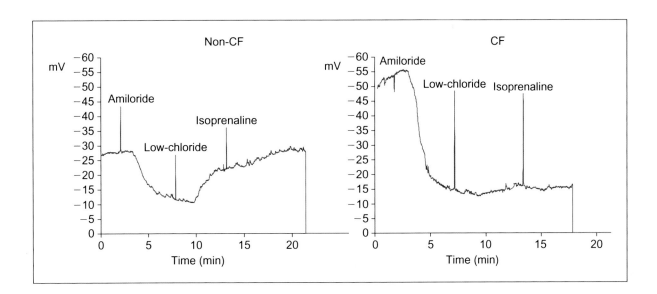

6.5 When compared with non-cystic fibrosis values, cystic fibrosis nasal PD is higher (more negative), more sensitive to inhibition with the Na^+ channel blocking agent, amiloride (both due to Na^+ hyperabsorption) and relatively insensitive to agents which induce Cl^- secretion (low chloride solutions and CFTR stimulation with the cyclic adenosine monophosphate agonist, isoprenaline) (courtesy of Dr Nick Simmonds).

were clearest early in life, at the time when growth (including that of head circumference) is at its most rapid. Screening has recently been introduced into the UK; there will be false positives, which will engender unnecessary anxiety, and false negatives, which may result in complacency. The balance of evidence is clearly in favour of population screening for CF so that early treatment can be given, and antenatal diagnosis offered for future pregnancies.

Clinical disease

Disease phenotype is variable; both the presentation (*Table 6.3*) and clinical course can differ greatly between individuals.

Respiratory disease

Respiratory disease is the main burden for patients, in terms of therapies (both prophylaxis and treatment), morbidity and ultimately mortality (>90% will die of respiratory failure). It is a common presenting feature in childhood, with recurrent cough, wheeze or frank pneumonia;

occasionally, children will be misdiagnosed as, for example, 'asthma' and will present with advanced features of disease such as chest deformity, finger clubbing (**6.6**) and significant bronchiectasis (**6.7**).

Lung (or, more accurately, airways) disease is characterized by early-onset bacterial infection and exaggerated and sustained neutrophilic inflammation; which comes first and

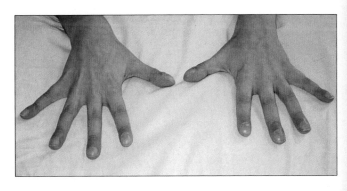

6.6 Finger clubbing.

Table 6.3 Presentations of cystic fibrosis by age group

Age group	Presenting complaint
Antenatal	• Chorionic villous sampling (known at-risk couple) • Foetal hyperechogenic bowel • Ultrasound diagnosis of bowel perforation
At or soon after birth	• Bowel obstruction (meconium ileus, bowel atresia) • Haemorrhagic disease of the newborn • Prolonged jaundice • Screening (population based or previously affected sibling)
Infancy and childhood	• Recurrent respiratory infections • Diarrhoea/steatorrhoea and failure to thrive • Rectal prolapse • Nasal polyps • Acute pancreatitis (PS patients only) • Portal hypertension and variceal haemorrhage • Pseudo-Bartter's syndrome, electrolyte abnormality • Hypoproteinaemia and oedema • Screening as a result of cystic fibrosis diagnosis in a sibling/relative
Adolescence and adult life	• Recurrent respiratory infections • Atypical asthma • Bronchiectasis • Male infertility (congenital bilateral absence of the vas deferens) • Electrolyte disturbance/heat exhaustion • Screening as a result of diagnosis in affected relative • Portal hypertension and variceal haemorrhage

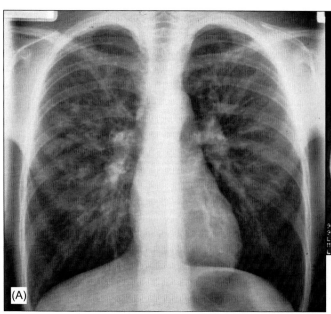
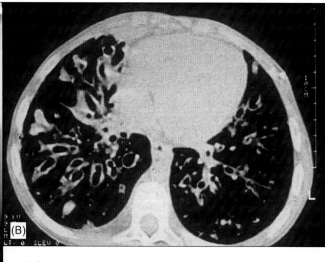

6.7 Severe, extensive bronchiectasis on chest X-ray (A) and computed tomography scan (B).

the exact relationship between the two remain uncertain. Several studies appear to show inflammatory changes preceding infection, whereas others do not. It is clear, however, that disease begins early and often in the absence of symptoms as demonstrated by both invasive and non-invasive (physiological) tests. The CF airway becomes infected with a rather narrow range of bacterial pathogens (*Table 6.4*). Fungi are relatively common, particularly *Aspergillus fumigatus*, although the main problem stems from an IgE-mediated immune response to the presence of these organisms within the airway rather than infection *per se*. Allergic bronchopulmonary aspergillosis should be considered in the context of an increase in airway obstruction and/or new chest X-ray changes (typically wedge-shaped shadows that may 'flit' or change frequently (**6.8**)), in particular if there is no response to intravenous antibiotics (*Table 6.5*). Non-tuberculous mycobacteria may be detected in asymptomatic individuals; it can often be difficult to determine whether these are pathogenic or not. Multiple isolates and new symptoms or those that fail to respond to conventional treatment would raise suspicion. CT findings that are useful in patients without CF (pulmonary nodules, peripheral mucus plugging) are so common in CF that interpretation is difficult. Treatment is most commonly with multiple antimycobacterial agents for prolonged periods of

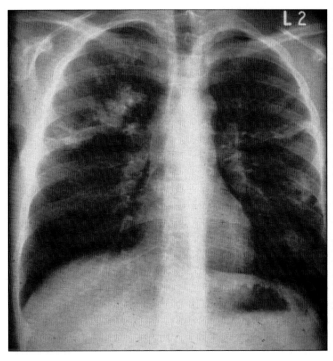

6.8 *Aspergillus fumigatus* hyphae stained with silver. Note the typical branching pattern of the fungal hyphae. (B) Allergic bronchopulmonary aspergillosis in the right upper lobe. Allergic bronchopulmonary aspergillosis is characterized radiologically by focal (often wedge-shaped), flitting areas of consolidation. The typical 'gloved finger' appearance is apparent.

Table 6.4 Pathogens commonly encountered in cystic fibrosis

Common	Rarer
Staphylococcus aureus (including, less commonly, MRSA)	*Achromobacter (Alcaligenes) xylosoxidans*
Haemophilus influenzae	*Inquilinus limosus*
Pseudomonas aeruginosa	*Ralstonia* sp.
Stenotrophomonas maltophilia	*Pandoraea* sp.
Burkholderia cepacia complex	*Acinetobacter baumannii*
Atypical mycobacteria	Other fungi, e.g. *Scedosporium* sp.
Aspergillus fumigatus	

Table 6.5 Major criteria for the diagnosis of allergic bronchopulmonary aspergillosis

Reversible bronchoconstriction	Blood eosinophilia
Pulmonary infiltrate(s)	Raised total serum IgE
Positive immediate skin-prick test	Positive IgG precipitins
Positive specific IgE (RAST)	Central bronchiectasis

Minor criteria include positive sputum culture, late skin test reaction and brown plugs in sputum.

RAST, radioallergosorbent test.

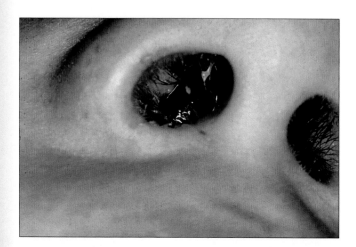

6.9 Large right-sided nasal polyp.

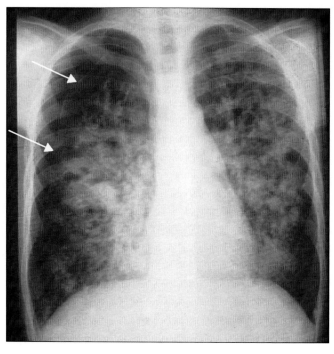

6.10 Right-sided pneumothorax (arrows) in a patient with severe cystic fibrosis lung disease.

time and thus is not embarked upon lightly. Other respiratory problems include nasal polyps (**6.9**), which often recur after surgical removal, and chronic sinusitis. Advanced respiratory disease can be complicated by severe haemoptysis (from hypertrophied bronchial vessels) and pneumothorax (**6.10**), either of which may present as an acute emergency.

Treatment of respiratory disease

Physiotherapy to aid the removal of secretions is the mainstay of treatment. Young children will usually be prescribed prophylactic anti-staphylococcal antibiotics orally; fears relating to increased risk of *Pseudomonas aeruginosa* acquisition appear to be limited to oral cephalosporins only. Regular surveillance with sputum culture or cough swabs should be employed and new organisms treated appropriately. First isolation of *P. aeruginosa* is usually eradicable if caught early and treated aggressively with a combination of systemic and topical (nebulized) antibiotics. Unfortunately, most patients ultimately become chronically infected with this organism, which assumes a mucoid phenotype (**6.11**) and becomes more difficult to treat; long-term suppressive treatment with nebulized antibiotics has been shown to be of benefit. Most patients acquire bacterial pathogens from the environment rather than other patients, but reports of highly transmissible strains of *P. aeruginosa* and *Burkholderia cepacia* complex organisms have led to strict infection control practices, including patient segregation in many clinics. Exacerbations of respiratory disease are treated with either oral or intravenous antibiotics depending on severity; multiple courses of the latter will often require the insertion of a semi-permanent intravenous access device such as a portacath (**6.12**). Adjuncts to treatment include mucolytic agents such as recombinant human DNase and hypertonic saline. Anti-inflammatory drugs are largely confined to research studies at present, although ibuprofen is widely used outside the UK. Azithromycin, one of the macrolide groups of antibiotics, is of benefit and may be working as an anti-inflammatory agent. Unfortunately, despite great improvements in lung function and survival over recent decades, most patients will develop bronchiectasis and respiratory failure; at this stage, transplantation is an option, although is limited by availability of organs and increased rates of obliterative bronchiolitis in children. However, for most, prognosis has substantially improved over the last few decades; median life expectancy has risen from under 10 years in the 1960s to an estimate of 40 years for babies born today (**6.13**).

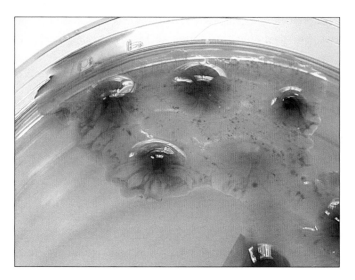

6.11 Mucoid *Pseudomonas aeruginosa*.

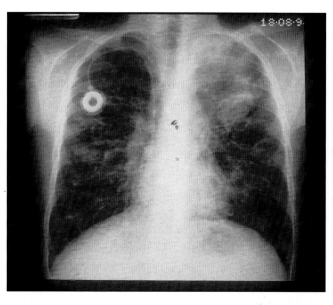

6.12 Radiological appearance of port positioned subcutaneously on right anterior chest wall; the catheter is inserted into the right subclavian vein, from where it enters the superior vena cava. Note there is severe, bilateral cystic fibrosis lung disease.

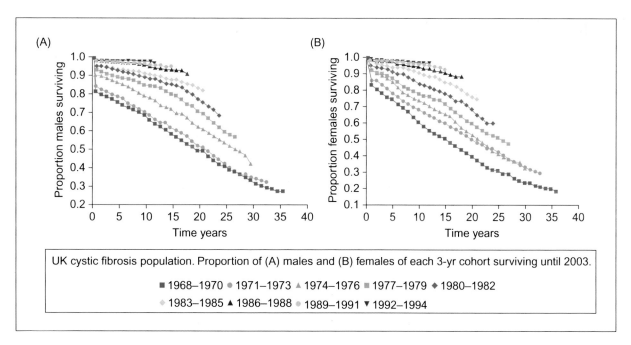

UK cystic fibrosis population. Proportion of (A) males and (B) females of each 3-yr cohort surviving until 2003.

■ 1968–1970 ● 1971–1973 ▲ 1974–1976 ■ 1977–1979 ◆ 1980–1982
◆ 1983–1985 ▲ 1986–1988 ● 1989–1991 ▼ 1992–1994

6.13 Survival curves for different birth cohorts of patients with cystic fibrosis in the UK (reproduced with permission from: Dodge JA, Lewis PA, Stanton M, Wilsher J. Cystic fibrosis mortality and survival in the UK: 1947–2003. *Eur Respir J* 2007; 29: 522–6. Epub 2006 Dec 20).

Gastrointestinal disease

Approximately 85–90% of patients with CF have exocrine pancreatic insufficiency; this results in malabsorption (particularly of fat), steatorrhoea, abdominal distension and failure to thrive; poor weight gain occurs first, but if left untreated, linear growth will also suffer. Stool elastase is low, most often undetectable. Pancreatic enzymes will be prescribed and the dose should be tapered to the dietary intake. The total lipase dose should be kept if possible to 10–15 000 lipase units/kg body weight/day. These are usually highly effective, although their efficacy can be enhanced if required with antacid drugs, such as H_2 agonists or proton pump inhibitors. Fat-soluble vitamins are also administered, including vitamin K, which has been shown to offer some protection against osteoporosis. Supplemental calories can be administered as high-calorie drinks, but if this fails to meet nutritional demands and weight gain is suboptimal, enteral feeding via a gastrostomy (**6.14**) may be required. Approximately 10% of infants with CF present shortly after birth with abdominal distension and bile-stained vomiting due to meconium ileus. The abdominal X-ray may show distended loops of bowel, an almost gas-free abdomen or free gas indicating perforation (**6.15**). In the absence of a complication such as perforation, a gastrograffin enema may relieve the obstruction, but some babies require surgery and even bowel resection. Patients with CF are also prone to subacute bowel obstruction due to inspissation of malabsorbed material in the terminal ileum and caecum, termed 'distal intestinal obstruction syndrome' or DIOS, a condition not seen in other malabsorptive conditions. It presents with colicky abdominal pain, constipation and abdominal distension. Acute treatment is with oral gastrograffin or intestinal lavage with balanced electrolyte solution; very rarely, surgery is needed. The differential diagnosis includes simple constipation, which may be severe in CF. Rectal prolapse may be the presenting feature and should always alert one to the possibility of CF; it can be a recurrent problem.

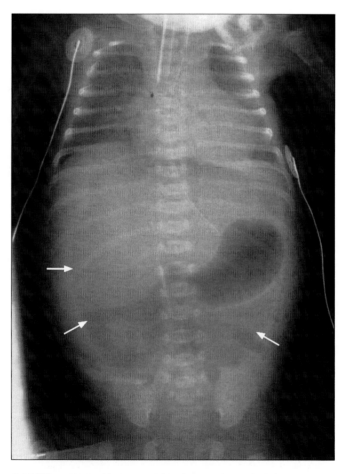

6.14 Gastrostomy button (child has also had an open Nissen's fundoplication); normally, the gastrostomy would be placed endoscopically.

6.15 Dilated bowel loops and free intraperitoneal air (arrows) in a child with perforated meconium ileus.

Liver disease

The characteristic abnormality is a focal biliary cirrhosis (**6.16**, **6.17**), which usually presents as hepatosplenomegaly detected at a routine clinical examination, or variceal haemorrhage. Abnormal liver function tests are common and non-specific; suspected CF liver disease should be investigated with ultrasound. Treatment is usually with ursodeoxycholic acid, although there is little evidence in support of this.

Other complications

CF-related diabetes is increasingly common in adolescence and adult life and is generally associated with a worse prognosis, in particular in females. It should be considered in patients with deteriorating nutritional status or poorer than expected lung function, even in the absence of the specific symptoms such as polyuria. It should be confirmed with glucose tolerance testing and/or a period of home blood glucose monitoring, and treated, in most cases, with insulin. Dietary management is completely different from that of juvenile-onset diabetes. A high-calorie, high-fat diet should be continued (unlike the diet recommended for type 1 diabetes mellitus alone), and insulin dosage adjusted to maintain good glycaemic control.

The majority of males with CF have congenital absence of the vas deferens leading to azospermia and infertility; older boys can undergo semen analysis to confirm this. CF bone disease is being increasingly recognized; risk factors include severe pulmonary involvement, inadequate nutrition and the use of systemic corticosteroids; patients are being

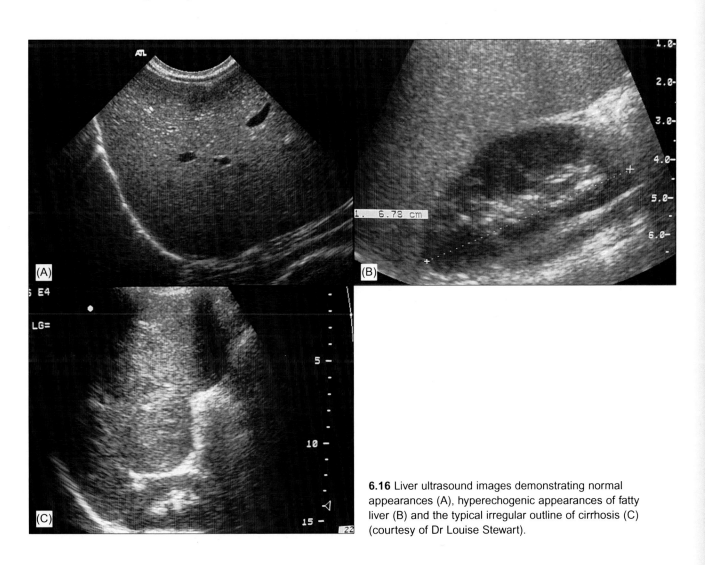

6.16 Liver ultrasound images demonstrating normal appearances (A), hyperechogenic appearances of fatty liver (B) and the typical irregular outline of cirrhosis (C) (courtesy of Dr Louise Stewart).

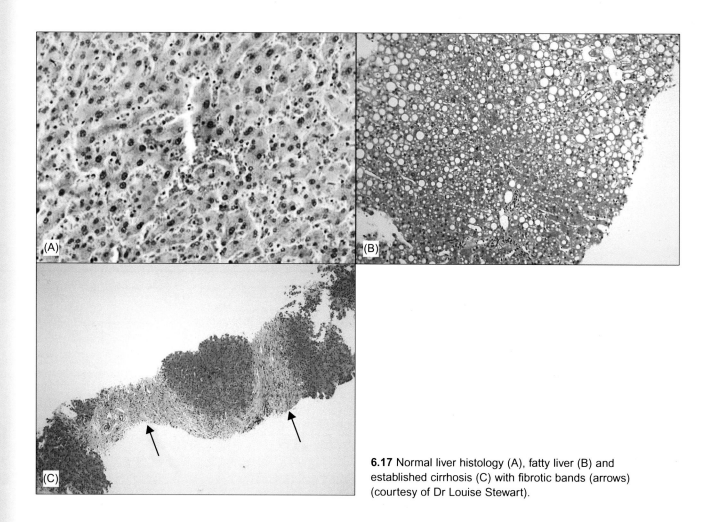

6.17 Normal liver histology (A), fatty liver (B) and established cirrhosis (C) with fibrotic bands (arrows) (courtesy of Dr Louise Stewart).

increasingly treated with vitamin K, which has proved useful in preventing this complication.

Further reading

Boucher RC. Airway surface dehydration in cystic fibrosis: pathogenesis and therapy. *Annu Rev Med* 2007; 58: 57–70.

Boyle MP. Update on maintaining bone health in cystic fibrosis. *Curr Opin Pulm Med* 2006; 12: 453–8.

Colombo C, Russo MC, Zazzeron L, Romano G. Liver disease in cystic fibrosis. *J Pediatr Gastroenterol Nutr* 2006; 43(Suppl 1): S49–55.

Ratjen F. What's new in CF airway inflammation: an update. *Paediatr Respir Rev* 2006; 7(Suppl 1): S70–2.

Rowe SM, Clancy JP. Advances in cystic fibrosis therapies. *Curr Opin Pediatr* 2006; 18: 604–13.

Wood DM, Smyth AR. Antibiotic strategies for eradicating Pseudomonas aeruginosa in people with cystic fibrosis. *Cochrane Database Syst Rev* 2006; (1): CD004197.

Chapter 7

Non-cystic fibrosis bronchiectasis

Mark A. Chilvers, Fiona Dickinson, Chris O'Callaghan

Introduction

Bronchiectasis describes a pathological state of the conducting airways manifested by radiographic evidence of bronchial dilatation and clinically by chronic productive cough. It is the end result of a number of pulmonary insults and predisposing conditions that injure the airways, leading eventually to recurrent or persistent airway infection and destruction.

Historically, bronchiectasis was common following childhood respiratory tract infections such as pertussis, tuberculosis and complicated measles. With the advent of immunization programmes and appropriate antibiotic usage over the last 40 years, incidence has declined greatly. However, recent improvements in diagnostic testing, using high-resolution computed tomography (HRCT) scanning of the chest, are uncovering more cases.

The true incidence of childhood bronchiectasis is unknown but varies between developed and developing nations (*Table 7.1*). Higher incidences are observed in communities where there is inadequate nutrition, crowded housing and poor hygiene.

Two studies have examined the incidence of childhood bronchiectasis in the UK. The first study reviewed 4000 children referred over an 8-year period for respiratory symptoms to a tertiary respiratory centre. They found that 1% were diagnosed with non-cystic fibrosis (non-CF) bronchiectasis (Nikolaizik, 1994). More recently, Eastham and colleagues (2004) found a high prevalence of bronchiectasis diagnosed by HRCT in north-east England (*Table 7.1*). The numbers in this study were added to by the inclusion of at-risk groups such as transplant recipients. Worryingly, the time taken from initial symptoms to diagnosis is often considerable. In Eastham's study, the

median time interval between onset of respiratory symptoms and diagnosis was 3 years. It is likely that bronchiectasis is still significantly underdiagnosed during childhood.

Pathogenesis

When an airway obstruction or infection is resolved in a timely fashion, there appears to be little effect on the airway. However, if an airway is obstructed, secretions will build up behind the obstruction. If these become infected, damage to the bronchial wall occurs. It is this combination that is thought most likely to cause bronchiectasis. Persistent and exaggerated inflammation (including increased neutrophil elastase, tumour necrosis factor α, interleukin 8 and 6) is present in bronchiectasis, which, together with a reduction in antiproteinases, contribute to the destruction of the elastic and muscular components of bronchial walls. The contractile forces of the surrounding lungs may contribute to the dilatation of the damaged airways.

Bronchiectasis can be classified radiologically and pathologically into three distinct groups.

1. *Cylindrical*: bronchi are minimally dilated with a straight regular outline and end squarely and abruptly.
2. *Varicose*: bronchi are dilated and interspersed by areas of relative constriction. The bronchi terminate with a bulbous and distorted end.
3. *Cystic or saccular*: bronchi become progressively more dilated and balloon-like. This dilatation increases as the bronchi approach the periphery of the lung. Air–fluid levels may be present.

Table 7.1 Global prevalence and incidence of non-cystic fibrosis bronchiectasis. The table highlights ethnic differences between countries and within ethnic subgroups. A higher incidence of bronchiectasis is observed in the New Zealand population. This is significantly higher in patients of Maori and Pacific descent. In contrast, a lower incidence is observed in Finnish children. Data for the UK are limited. Two studies have estimated prevalence. A study in 1963 estimated a UK prevalence of 1 in 10 000 (Clark, 1963); however, more recent data from 2004 suggest a much higher prevalence (Eastham, 2004)

Ethnic origin	Incidence/100 000	Prevalence	Year
New Zealand	3.7	1:3000	2005
Pacific	17.8	1:625	
Maori	4.8		
European	1.5		
Australia		5:1000	2002
Aborigines		15:1000	
Samoa		6:1000	1996
UK			
Newcastle	1.0	1:5800	2004
Scotland		1:10 000	1963
Finland	0.5		1998
Adult/Paediatric	3.9		1998
USA			
Adult/Paediatric		52:100 000	2004
Alaska		16:1000	2000

Data taken from: Chang 2003, Clark 1963, Eastham 2004, Redding 2004 and Twiss 2005

Bronchiectasis may be either focal (**7.1**) or diffuse (**7.2**). Focal bronchiectasis may follow a severe pneumonia, foreign body or localized intrinsic or extrinsic bronchial compression. Diffuse bronchiectasis suggests an underlying disorder that disrupts the mucociliary escalator (**7.3**). The loss of ciliary function results in mucus retention, infection and epithelial destruction. As the epithelium regenerates it forms cuboidal and squamous epithelium. From here, the damaged airway progresses through distinct stages of bronchiectatic development. First, cylindrical bronchiectasis is characterized by focal destruction of elastic tissue, epithelial oedema and infiltration of inflammatory cells. As airway damage continues, the bronchus may become blocked by fibrous tissue, which contracts and results in the areas of airway constriction and dilatation observed in varicose bronchiectasis. Further disease progression results in damage extending into the muscle layer and cartilage to cause the cystic or saccular phase of bronchiectasis. Surrounding tissue becomes damaged and destruction to end arteries occurs. Revascularization with the formation of anastamoses between bronchial and pulmonary arteries has been observed around saccular bronchiectatic lung (*Table 7.2*). Saccular and varicose bronchiectasis are both considered irreversible, although cylindrical bronchiectasis may be reversible as the resolution of radiological changes has been observed following appropriate treatment (Eastham, 2004).

Table 7.2 Airway structural changes in respiratory disease. This summarizes the relative magnitude of histological changes observed in patients with bronchiectasis in comparison with asthma and chronic obstructive pulmonary disease (COPD). Patients with bronchiectasis have significant mucous gland hyperplasia with mild epithelial damage, angiogenesis and smooth muscle alteration (with permission from Bergeron and Boulet, 2006)

Variables	Asthma	Irritant-induced occupational asthma	COPD	Bronchiectasis
Mucous gland hyperplasia	++	++?	++++	+++
Subepithelial collagen deposition	+++	++++	+	+
Angiogenesis	+++	?	+	+
Increased smooth muscle	+++	++?	+	+
Increased proteoglycan deposition	+++	+++?	+	+
Increased elastin	++	++	?	+
Epithelial damage	+++	++++	++	+

Scores: +, mild; ++, moderate; +++, significant; ++++, marked; ?, uncertain.

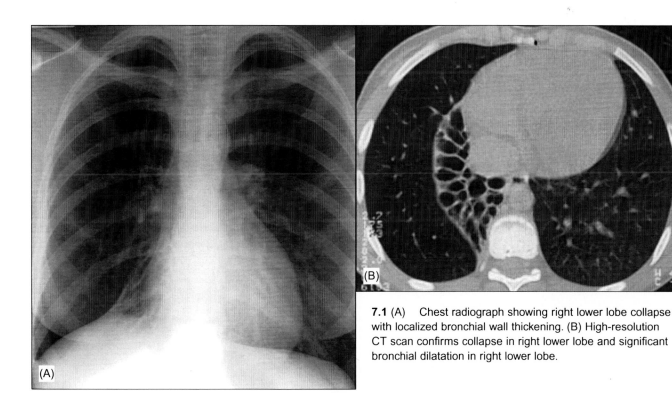

(A)

(B)

7.1 (A)   Chest radiograph showing right lower lobe collapse with localized bronchial wall thickening. (B) High-resolution CT scan confirms collapse in right lower lobe and significant bronchial dilatation in right lower lobe.

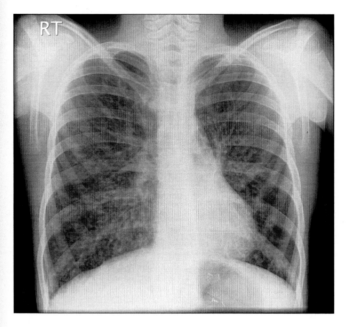

7.2 Extensive bronchial wall thickening with some parenchymal changes in a child who has had a Nissen's fundoplication for chronic aspiration. A degree of hyperinflation is also present.

Aetiology

A variety of different causes for non-CF bronchiectasis have been identified (*Table 7.3a,b*). These range from congenital lung abnormalities and immunological defects (discussed in Chapter 9) to chronic aspiration **(7.2)**. *Table 7.4* highlights that it is possible to identify an underlying aetiology in approximately 70% of cases assuming relevant diagnostic tests are available.

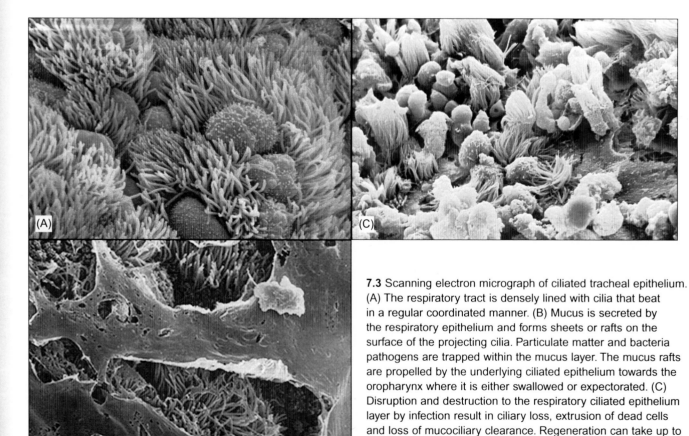

7.3 Scanning electron micrograph of ciliated tracheal epithelium. (A) The respiratory tract is densely lined with cilia that beat in a regular coordinated manner. (B) Mucus is secreted by the respiratory epithelium and forms sheets or rafts on the surface of the projecting cilia. Particulate matter and bacteria pathogens are trapped within the mucus layer. The mucus rafts are propelled by the underlying ciliated epithelium towards the oropharynx where it is either swallowed or expectorated. (C) Disruption and destruction to the respiratory ciliated epithelium layer by infection result in ciliary loss, extrusion of dead cells and loss of mucociliary clearance. Regeneration can take up to 12 weeks.

Table 7.3a Aetiology of non-cystic fibrosis bronchiectasis: respiratory and systemic conditions. Numerous congenital abnormalities have been described that result in bronchiectasis. Acquired insults range from aspiration, inhalation and postinfectious injuries, which may cause permanent damage. Underlying respiratory conditions have been reported to cause bronchiectasis. Systemic diseases can also result in non-cystic fibrosis bronchiectasis, notably inflammatory bowel disease

Congenital	• Broncho-arterial malformation • Bronchial atresia with bronchocoele/bronchogenic cyst • Cystic adenomatoid malformation • Lobar emphysema • Pulmonary artery sling • Hamartoma • Bronchomalacia/Williams-Campbell syndrome • Absent pulmonary valve syndrome • Tracheo-oesophageal fistula • Yellow nail syndrome • α1-antitrypsin deficiency
Respiratory	• Asthma/middle lobe syndrome • Primary ciliary dyskinesia • Bronchioloitis obliterans
Aspiration	• Palm oil • Foreign body • Severe neurological impairment; chronic aspiration
Inhalation injury	

Postinfection	• Adenovirus/respiratory syncitial virus
	• Measles
	• Pertussis
	• Tuberculosis
	• Mycoplasma
	• Varicella
	• Allergic bronchopulmonary aspergillosis
	• Pneumonia:
	   – Necrotizing
	   – Unknown cause

Gastrointestinal	• Chronic gastro-oesophageal reflux • Inflammatory bowel disease
Idiopathic	

Table 7.3b Immunological abnormalities. With a greater understanding and ability to readily investigate the immune system, a large variety of immunological defects have been described which result in non-CF bronchiectasis. In addition, it is important to exclude secondary immune defects.

PRIMARY IMMUNE DEFECTS

B-cell deficiency
- Panhypogammaglobulinaemia
- Common variable immune deficiency
- Undefined combined immunodeficiency
- IgA deficiency
- IgG deficiency
- X-linked agammaglobulinaemia
- Qualitative antibody deficiency

T-cell deficiency
- Hyper IgM syndrome
- MHC class 2 deficiency
- Severe combined immunodeficiency
- Ataxia telangiectasia
- Wiscott-Aldrich syndrome

Phagocytic defects
- Hyper-IgE syndrome
- Chronic granulomatous disease

Complement
- Complement deficiency
- Mannose-binding protein deficiency

SECONDARY IMMUNE DEFECTS

- Human immunodeficiency virus
- Post radiotherapy/chemotherapy

Table 7.4 Frequency of aetiological abnormalities observed in non-cystic fibrosis bronchiectasis. Several series have evaluated the underlying aetiologies responsible for non-cystic fibrosis bronchiectasis. The table summarizes the percentage of cases caused by different pathological groups. It is possible to identify an underlying cause in up to 90% of patients presenting with bronchiectasis. Values are percentages of the total number of children in each reported series

Aetiology	Nikolaizik (1994) (%) $n = 41$	Eastham (2004) (%) $n = 93$	Li (2005) (%) $n = 136$	Dogru (2005) (%) $n = 204$	Karadag (2005) (%) $n = 136$	Twiss (2005) (%) $n = 65$
Congenital lung abnormality	15	9	4	2	3	
Primary ciliary dyskinesia	17	1	15	12	6	
Immunological:						
Total	27	20	31	6	15	17
Primary	20		29	5		6
Secondary	7		4	1		11
Idiopathic	7	18	26	49	38	54
Aspiration	5	5	18	3	4	6
Postinfectious	29	30	4	16	30	22
Secondary respiratory disorder		10		12	4	
Other		7				

Bronchiectasis following infection (e.g. *Bordetella pertussis* or *Mycobacterium tuberculosis*) is much less common in the current era, with improved standards of living, immunization and access to medical care. Primary or secondary immunological defects are now commonly observed as a cause of childhood bronchiectasis. Chronic or acute severe aspiration is responsible for a proportion of cases. Primary ciliary dyskinesia has been reported as an underlying cause of non-CF bronchiectasis in up to 15% of patients (**7.4, 7.5**). This condition may be under-reported due to a lack of centres offering a reliable diagnostic service. Diagnosis of primary ciliary dyskinesia is difficult and often results in late diagnosis. Secondary changes to ciliary structure and function are commonly seen following an upper respiratory tract infection and make interpretation difficult.

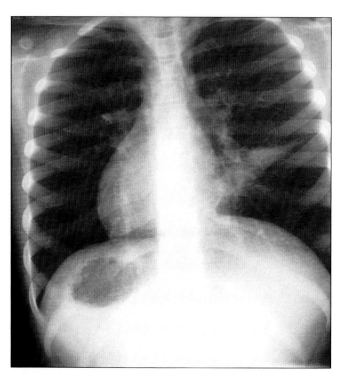

7.4 Situs inversus with mirror image left middle lobe consolidation. This patient was later diagnosed with primary ciliary dyskinesia.

Symptoms and signs

The most common symptom is a chronic cough, which is invariably wet sounding and can be productive. Mild haemoptysis may occur in between 4% and 14% of patients. Fever, however, is uncommon at presentation being, reported in only 8% of children (Dagli, 2000; Dogru, 2005).

In young children with bronchiectasis, a diagnosis may be delayed for several reasons: they are usually unable to expectorate sputum even when they have a wet cough; children usually remain afebrile despite ongoing chronic lung inflammation and infection; even in the presence of bronchiectasis, chest auscultation is usually normal, and in young children it is difficult to perform objective lung function testing such as spirometry. Therefore, a persistent wet sounding cough may be the only feature of bronchiectasis in the paediatric population. Symptoms often begin in the preschool years; children with non-CF bronchiectasis are most likely to have symptoms of wheezing and a productive cough for at least a year before diagnosis and 40% of newly diagnosed adult bronchiectatic patients report symptoms that began at less than 10 years of age (Redding, 2004; Pasteur, 2000).

Clinical examination may reveal a chest deformity including Harrison's sulci, lordosis and hyperinflation. Finger clubbing may be observed. Auscultatory findings are usually localized to bronchiectatic areas and include crackles and wheeze. Nasal inspection may reveal rhinorrhoea or polyps. Other features observed might include skin lesions and hepatosplenomegaly if underlying immunodeficiency is a feature. Failure to thrive may often be seen in any child with a significant chronic illness.

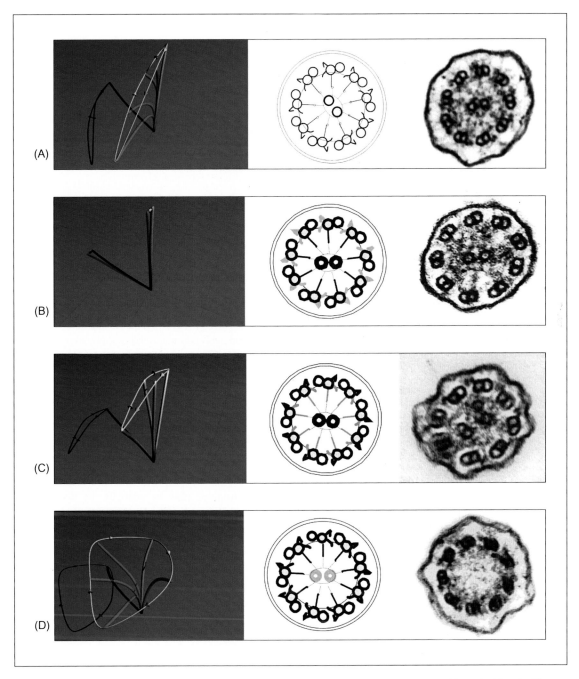

7.5 Ciliary beat pattern and ultrastructural abnormalities found in patients with primary ciliary dyskinesia. The three-dimensional diagrams illustrate the different beat patterns in patients with primary ciliary dyskinesia (adapted from Chilvers *et al*, 2003). The diagram shows the classical '9+2' ultrastructural arrangement. Light shaded areas correspond to the missing structural components on the transmission electron micrograph in the right-hand column. (A) A normal planar beat pattern with a forward backward 'whip-like' motion. This is observed in normal cilia with a classical '9+2' ultrastructural arrangement. (B) A stiff immotile beat pattern seen in patients with a defect of outer dynein arms or both outer and inner dynein arms. (C) A stiff planar beat pattern seen in patients with either a defect of the radial spoke and inner dynein arms or inner dynein arms alone. (D) A large gyrating beat pattern seen in patients with ciliary transposition defect.

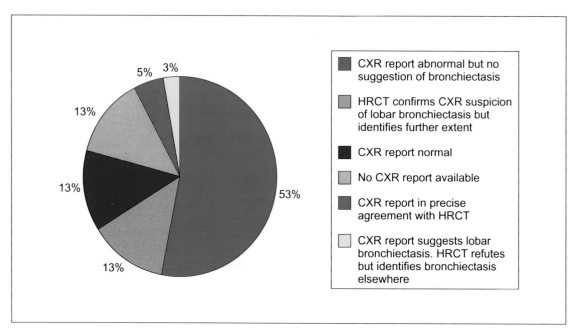

7.6 Radiological agreement between chest radiograph and high-resolution computed tomography for children diagnosed with non-cystic fibrosis bronchiectasis (with permission from Eastham, 2004).

Diagnosis

Knowing the underlying diagnosis is important as this may significantly influence patient management. Suspicion should come from a detailed history and occasionally from physical examination. A chest radiograph may be normal in up to 50% of patients with bronchiectasis demonstrated bronchographically, particularly in the early stages of disease (Currie, 1987). Eastham found that only 5% of chest radiographs agreed with HRCT findings in children with non-CF bronchiectasis and 50% did not suggest a diagnosis of bronchiectasis (**7.6**).

As the disease progresses, radiographic changes start to become evident. These may simply be the findings of lobar collapse (**7.1**). More specific appearances include parallel line opacities (tram tracks) due to thickened dilated bronchi. As these become fluid-filled, bronchocoeles/tubular opacities (ladies fingers) may be seen. If the abnormal bronchi are viewed end on then ring lesions are seen. Cystic lesions are a finding in late advanced bronchiectasis. The lower lobes are most commonly affected.

Historically, the gold standard for diagnosis of bronchiectasis was a bronchogram (**7.7, 7.8**). However, this is invasive, uncomfortable and may underestimate the severity of the disease. It has now been superseded by HRCT, which is highly accurate with sensitivity and specificity greater than 90% (Edwards, 2004).

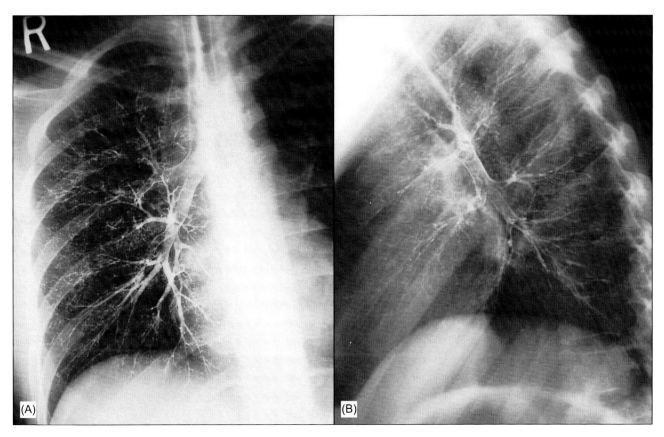

7.7 A bronchogram of a healthy subject. This illustrates normal calibre bronchi that exhibit a gradual tapering as they extend to the peripheries of the lung fields.

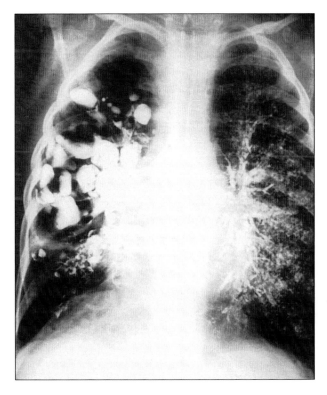

7.8 A bronchogram showing extensive right-sided cystic bronchiectasis.

With HRCT, the criteria for the diagnosis of bronchiectasis include dilatation of bronchi as determined by a bronchial lumen/adjacent pulmonary artery ratio of greater than 1 (signet ring sign), parallel bronchial walls with lack of peripheral tapering (tramline sign) and visualization of bronchi in the outer 1–2 cm of the lung (**7.9–7.11**). HRCT will demonstrate extent and severity of bronchiectasis but it is not useful in helping to identify an underlying cause, which must be actively sought.

Investigations are led by the history and examination findings. For patients where the cause is unclear, we undertake basic investigations and follow the patient regularly adding investigations as appropriate. For example, at the first visit, investigations would include: a sweat test; CF genotype; basic immunological tests (immunoglobulins and subclasses; functional specific antibody responses and complement); full blood count; α_1-antitrypsin levels; standard culture of respiratory pathogens from sputum and liquid culture to look for atypical mycobacterium; quantiferon and Mantoux tests to help rule out TB. We have a low threshold for bronchoscopy and bronchoalveolar lavage to evaluate airway structure and to obtain secretions for culture. A pH study can be conveniently arranged at the same time with the probe inserted under anaesthetic following bronchoscopy. In a patient with chronic nasal symptoms, ciliary functional studies and electron microscopy will be performed. Measurement of nasal nitric oxide is a

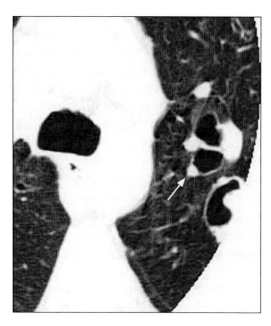

7.9 Signet ring sign in marked cystic bronchiectasis (arrow); bronchial diameter exceeds that of adjacent vessel and bronchi visible in the outer 1–2 cm of the lung.

useful screening test for patients suspected of primary ciliary dyskinesia but requires cooperation, which precludes its use with young children.

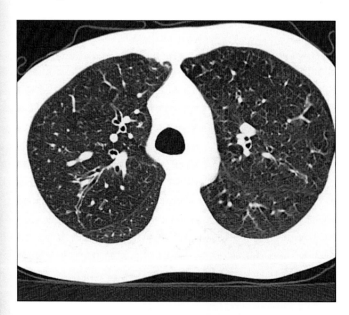

7.10 Bronchiectasis demonstrated in the right lung by lack of normal tapering of a bronchus as it approaches the periphery.

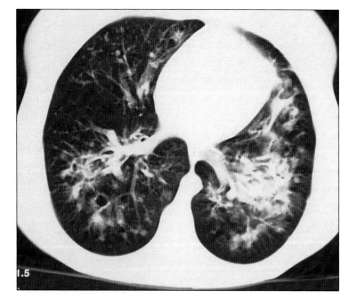

7.11 High-resolution computed tomography showing extensive cystic bronchiectasis in an adolescent girl. Evidence of retained fluid and fluid levels and peripheral bronchial impaction.

Management

Patients should be managed by a paediatrician with a respiratory interest and may require shared care from a tertiary centre. Management is similar to that of CF (see Chapter 6) (*Table 7.5*). Regular review of patients with sputum culture and pulmonary function testing is mandatory. Left untreated there will be disease progression; however, with appropriate treatment, patients can do very well. In children and adults with primary ciliary dyskinesia, unlike those with CF, once a diagnosis was made and intensive respiratory management was initiated, lung function was preserved during 15 years of follow-up (**7.12**).

Treatment for bronchiectasis remains primarily medical. Therapy is targeted at airway clearance and aggressive elimination of infection. Antibiotic treatment should be

Table 7.5 Management of non-cystic fibrosis bronchiectasis. The management follows similar lines to that for cystic fibrosis. Aggressive antibiotic use together with a daily physiotherapy routine are important. Regular microbiological surveillance and pulmonary function testing are needed to monitor disease progression and therapeutic intervention. It is important to ensure that patients are fully immunized. Surgical intervention is now uncommon with aggressive medical management. However, it may be required for localised disease, failure of medical therapy and massive haemoptysis. Recurrent haemoptysis may require bronchial artery embolisation.

Antibiotics	• Treat upper respiratory tract infections • Intravenous in acute exacerbations • Nebulized/oral prophylaxis
Physiotherapy	• Daily therapy; increased in exacerbations • Promote exercise
Airway inflammation	• Inhaled bronchodilators/corticosteroids
Microbiological surveillance	• Identify acute infection • Direct antibiotic therapy • Prevent bacterial colonization • Infection control
Pulmonary function testing	• Monitor disease progression • Identify respiratory exacerbation • Evaluate treatment response
Immunization	• Annual influenza vaccination • Pneumococcal vaccination
Nutrition	• Promote adequate lung growth
Psychosocial	• Access to economic entitlements • Patient support groups, e.g. primary ciliary dyskinesia family support group
Pulmonary artery embolization	• Recurrent/persistent haemoptysis
Surgery	• Localized resectable disease • Localized disease causing severe symptoms/infection not responding to medical treatment • Abscess formation • Life-threatening bleeding/haemoptysis

directed against the common infecting organisms in non-CF bronchiectasis, *Streptococcus pneumoniae* and *Haemophilus influenzae*, and used in acute and chronic exacerbating stages of infection. A low threshold for intravenous therapy may be indicated to minimize lung destruction. *Pseudomonas aeruginosa* is uncommon in non-CF bronchiectasis in children, but is associated with a decline in lung function and so should be aggressively eradicated in a similar fashion to that employed in CF (Chapter 6).

If there is an underlying asthmatic component, inhaled corticosteroids and bronchodilators may be of benefit, but use should be correlated with pulmonary function

measurements. Annual vaccination against influenza is required. Further vaccination against pneumococcus may be required if not routinely vaccinated or found to have a poor immunological response when tested.

Chest physiotherapy and postural drainage assist in the mobilization of endobronchial secretions. This should be performed regularly and increased at times of infective exacerbations. Exercise should be encouraged. The role of nebulized recombinant DNase and hypertonic saline remain speculative in non-CF bronchiectasis.

With earlier detection and improved medical treatment, invasive therapies (*Table 7.5*) are rarely needed. Children may have significant morbidity from recurrent haemoptysis, which may require bronchial artery embolization. Studies of surgical intervention, such as excision of localized disease, have reported good outcomes.

Prognosis

Paediatric data on disease progression and mortality are limited. Studies have reported annual rates of decline in forced expiratory volume in 1 second (FEV_1) from 1.5% to 3% per annum, which is dependent on the presence of chronic infection, notably *Pseudomonas aeruginosa* and *Haemophilus influenzae* (Angrill, 2002). In general, the rate

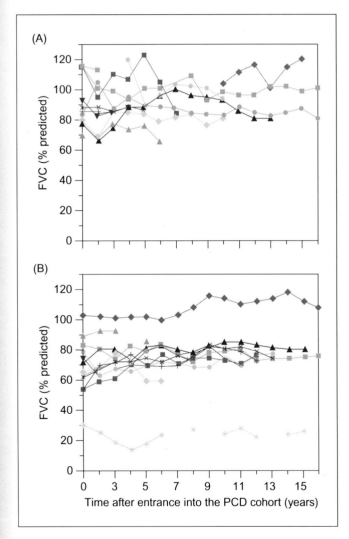

7.12 Forced vital capacity (FVC) % predicted in children (A) and adults (B) with primary ciliary dyskinesia (PCD). The data illustrate that, with appropriate management, lung function can be maintained over a 15-year period with little decline (with permission from Ellerman *et al*, 1997).

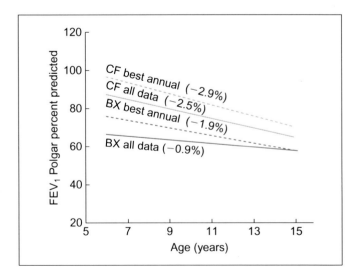

7.13 Model to show estimated decline in FEV_1 in children with non-cystic fibrosis bronchiectasis (BX) as compared with cystic fibrosis (CF) controls. The 'best annual' refers to the best FEV_1 value in that calendar year and 'all data' uses all available data (with permission from Twiss *et al*, 2006).

of decline seems to be slower than that for patients with CF (**7.13**). Studies in CF have shown that patients with normal lung function may still have significant lung damage on more sensitive tests including HRCT and, thus, normal spirometry should be interpreted with caution.

Appropriate medical management can slow the rate of progression of the disease, and therefore early diagnosis and intervention are vital to minimize long-term morbidity and mortality.

Summary

- Non-CF bronchiectasis may be underdiagnosed in children.
- A child with a persistent moist sounding cough greater than 6–12 weeks' duration requires further evaluation.
- A chest radiograph may be normal in 50% of patients with non-CF bronchiectasis.
- Diagnosis is made by HRCT scan.
- In at least 70% of cases, there is an underlying aetiology, which should be actively sought.
- Aggressive medical management will slow disease progression and preserve lung function.

Acknowledgements

The authors would like to thank Mr Andrew Rutman for help in supplying some of the images used in this chapter.

Further reading

Angrill J, Agusti C, De Celis R, *et al.* Bronchial inflammation and colonisation in patients with clinically stable bronchiectasis. *Am J Respir Crit Care Med* 2001; 164: 1628–32.

Angrill J, Agusti C, de Celis R, *et al.* Bacterial colonisation in patients with bronchiectasis: microbiological pattern and risk factors. *Thorax* 2002; 57: 15–19.

Bergeron C, Boulet LP. Strutural changes in airway diseases: characteristics, mechanisms, consequences and pharmacological modulation. *Chest* 2006; 129: 1068–87.

Chang AB, Masel JP, Boyce NC, Wheaton G, Torzillo PJ. Non-CF bronchiectasis: clinical and HRCT evaluation. *Pediatr Pulmonol* 2003; 35: 477–83.

Chilvers MA, Rutman A, O'Callaghan C. Ciliary beat pattern is associated with specific ultrastructural defects in primary ciliary dyskinesia. *J Allergy Clin Immunol* 2003; 112: 518–24.

Clark NS. Bronchiectasis in childhood. *BMJ* 1963; 5323: 80–8.

Currie DC, Cooke JC, Morgan AD, *et al.* Interpretation of bronchograms and chest radiographs in patients with chronic sputum production. *Thorax* 1987; 42: 278–84.

Dagli E. Non cystic fibrosis bronchiectasis. *Paed Resp Rev* 2000; 1: 64–70.

Dogru D, Nik-Ain A, Kiper N, *et al.* Bronchiectasis: the consequence of late diagnosis in chronic respiratory symptoms. *J Trop Ped* 2005; 51: 362–5.

Eastham KM, Fall AJ, Mitchell L, Spencer DA. The need to redefine non-cystic fibrosis bronchiectasis in childhood. *Thorax* 2004; 59: 324–7.

Edwards EA, Metcalfe R, Milne DG, Thompson J, Byrnes CA. Retrospective review of children presenting with non cystic fibrosis bronchiectasis: HRCT features and clinical relationships. *Pediatr Pulmonol* 2003; 36: 87–93.

Ellerman A, Bisgaard H. Longitudinal study of lung function in a cohort of primary ciliary dyskinesia. *Eur Respir J* 1997; 10: 2376–9.

Karadag B, Karakoc F, Ersu R, Kut A, Bakac S, Dagli E. Non-Cystic Fibrosis bronchiectasis in children: a persisting problem in developing countries. *Respir* 2005; 72: 233–8.

Li AM, Sonnappa S, Lex C, *et al.* Non-CF bronchiectasis: does knowing the aetiology lead to changes in management? *Eur Respir J* 2005; 26: 8–14.

Nikolaizik WH, Warner JO. Aetiology of chronic supporative lung disease. *Arch Dis Child* 1994; 70: 141–2.

Pasteur MC, Helliwell SM, Houghton SJ, *et al.* An investigation into causative factors in patients with bronchiectasis. *Am J Respir Crit Care Med* 2000; 162: 1277–84.

Redding G, Singleton R, Lewis T, *et al.* Early radiographic and clinical features associated with bronchiectasis in children. *Pediatr Pulmonol* 2004; **37**: 297–304.

Spencer DA. From hemp seed to porcupine quill to HRCT: advances in the diagnosis and epidemiology of bronchiectasis. *Arch Dis Child*; 90: 712–4.

Twiss J, Metcalfe R, Edwards E, Byrnes C. New Zealand national incidence of bronchiectasis 'too high' for a developed country. *Arch Dis Child* 2005; 90: 737–40.

Twiss J, Stewart AW, Byrnes CA. Longitudinal pulmonary function of childhood bronchiectasis and comparison with cystic fibrosis. *Thorax* 2006; 61: 414–8.

Chapter 8

Reflux and aspiration

Ranjan Suri, Indra Narang

Introduction

Aspiration is an important cause of respiratory morbidity in children. Although it is more common in newborns, it continues to be a problem throughout childhood. Short-term manifestations include cough, wheeze, respiratory infections and atelectasis. Long-term consequences can be more serious and include bronchiectasis and chronic lung disease. This chapter reviews the aetiology and current approach to the diagnosis and management of aspiration and gastro-oesophageal reflux (GOR) in children.

Aetiology

Aspiration from above

The aspiration of nasal or sinus secretions, oropharyngeal contents, swallowed liquids or a foreign body is referred to as aspiration from above. Causes can be divided into congenital and acquired.

Congenital
- Developmental, e.g. prematurity, fatigue aspiration.
- Abnormal swallow
  - *Anatomical*: oesophageal atresia/tracheo-oesophageal fistula, laryngotracheal cleft, cleft palate, choanal atresia/stenosis, micrognathia, macroglossia, pharyngeal diverticulum, vascular rings/slings.
  - *Neuromuscular*: cerebral palsy, myopathies, myotonic dystrophy, Werdnig Hoffmann disease.
  - *Other syndromes*: familial dysautonomia, Mobius syndrome.

Acquired
- Anatomical anomalies: tracheostomy, palatopharyngeal incompetence.
- Functional, e.g. sinus disease.
- Foreign body aspiration.
- Respiratory illness causing increased work during breathing, e.g. acute bronchiolitis.

Aspiration from below

Aspiration of gastric contents into the airways is referred to as aspiration from below. It comprises a complex of disorders involving oesophageal dysmotility and GOR.

Oesophageal dysmotility
Disorders affecting the proximal oesophagus:

- Primary
  - cricopharyngeal hypotension, incoordination, achalasia
- Secondary
  - cerebral palsy
  - meningocoele
  - Arnold–Chiari malformation
  - familial dysautonomia
  - myasthenia gravis
  - muscular dystrophy
  - polymyositis.

Disorders affecting the distal oesophagus:

- Primary
  - achalasia
  - diffuse oesophageal spasm
  - non-specific oesophageal motility disorders

- Secondary
  - GOR
  - Hirschprung's disease
  - post-tracheo-oesophageal fistula repair
  - post-oesophageal atresia repair.

Gastro-oesophageal reflux

GOR is the involuntary passage of gastric contents into the oesophagus. It is a physiological event occurring in every individual several times a day. In the first months of life, it can present with regurgitation. 'Pathological GOR' occurs when the reflux episodes happen too frequently, when the clearance of the refluxate is poor, or symptoms other than regurgitation occur. It can be due to:

- decreased lower oesophageal sphincter pressure;
- a transient increase in intra-abdominal pressure that exceeds the resting level of lower oesophageal sphincter pressure.

The mechanism by which GOR causes respiratory illness in children is not completely understood. GOR is common in children, but is not always associated with respiratory illness. However, many children with chronic respiratory disease do have GOR. GOR can be either the cause or the end result of the respiratory disease. Alternatively, these may coexist but bear no relationship to each other.

Gastro-oesophageal reflux and aspiration causing respiratory disease

Direct effects of aspiration
These can be:

- *Tracheitis, pneumonia, atelectasis:* caused by airway inflammation by direct contact with the aspirated material.
- *Laryngospasm, bronchospasm:* caused by airway reflex from irritation of the upper airway.
- *Airway hyperreactivity:* secondary to airway inflammation from aspiration.

Indirect effects of gastro-oesophageal reflux
This can be reflex bronchoconstriction caused by oesophageal acidification without aspiration.

Respiratory disease causing gastro-oesophageal reflux and aspiration
- Hyperinflation and diaphragmatic flattening with secondary stretching of the crura.
- Changes in abdominopleural pressure gradient: caused by negative intrathoracic pressure and increased abdominal pressure, e.g. when coughing.
- Effects of medication (e.g. caffeine) causing decreased lower oesophageal sphincter pressure.

Disorders associated with gastro-oesophageal reflux
GOR is prevalent in patients suffering from a pre-existing respiratory illness. These include the following:

- chronic lung disease of prematurity
- oesophageal atresia/tracheo-oesophageal fistula
- congenital diaphragmatic hernia
- hiatus hernia
- failure to thrive
- apnoea
- cystic fibrosis
- asthma
- neurological/neuromuscular disorders.

Presentation

GOR and aspiration can present in a number of different ways. Often they are not clearly defined in the history, as young children with aspiration may not exhibit overt findings of inability to swallow or vomiting. They may have silent aspiration and have findings of only increased respiratory symptoms, e.g. respiratory mucus, chronic cough, wheeze.

The modes of presentation of a child with aspiration include the following.

Common
- Chronic cough: associated with feeding and swallowing, night-time cough; may be misdiagnosed as cough-variant asthma.
- Gagging, choking with feeds.
- Increased respiratory mucus and congestion.
- Vomiting.
- Refusal to feed: may be associated with GOR.
- Wheezing.
- Recurrent pneumonia/bronchiectasis.

- Recurrent otitis media/sinusitis: due to nasal reflux, e.g. cleft palate.
- Oesophagitis.
- Abnormal arching (hyperextension) of the head, neck, and thorax (Sandifer syndrome).

Less common
- Apnoea or acute life-threatening event.
- Failure to thrive: inadequate intake due to painful swallowing
- Stridor or hoarseness: inflammation and oedema of the pharynx/vocal cords.
- Dental erosion: night-time acid reflux bathing the posterior dentition.
- Anaemia, haemoptysis, melaena: severe haemorrhagic oesophagitis.
- Pulmonary fibrosis: chronic inflammation of the airways and lung parenchyma.
- Bronchiolitis obliterans.

Diagnostic investigations

Aspiration
The following can provide diagnostic information on aspiration:

- chest radiograph
- videofluoroscopy
- tube oesophagram
- laryngotracheobronchoscopy and bronchoalveolar lavage
- high-resolution computed tomography scan of the chest.

Chest radiograph
A chest X-ray can be useful in diagnosing aspiration (8.1). However, a normal chest X-ray does not exclude the condition.

Videofluoroscopy
Videofluoroscopy provides the best imaging of swallowing. This study will assess the competence of suck in the infant and swallow in the older child, and therefore should ideally be performed under the observation of a paediatric speech and language therapist. Significant swallowing dysfunction (8.2) may lead to aspiration and can occur in infants

who do not have evidence of GOR, feeding difficulties or neurological problems.

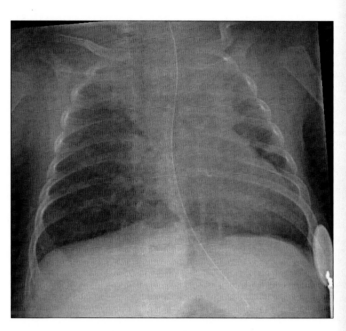

8.1 A 2-month-old, nasogastrically fed infant who presented with recurrent respiratory distress, cough and a persistent oxygen requirement. A pH study confirmed severe gastro-oesophageal reflux. The chest X-ray shows bilateral upper lobe opacification secondary to aspiration.

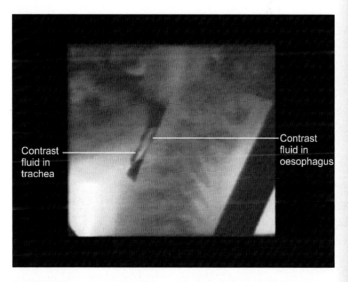

8.2 Videofluoroscopy showing aspiration of contrast fluid into the trachea. This patient had a history of recurrent respiratory tract infections secondary to aspiration caused by swallowing incoordination and weakness.

Tube oesophagram

A tube oesophagram will provide sufficient structural detail of the upper gastrointestinal tract to aid in the diagnosis of structural defects, such as tracheo-oesophageal fistula (**8.3**), which may be the cause of or contribute to aspiration into the lung.

Laryngotracheobronchoscopy and bronchoalveolar lavage

Direct vision of the upper and lower airways may be helpful in assessing malacia, which is associated with an increased risk of GOR, and to look for structural defects contributing to aspiration, such as tracheo-oesophageal fistula and laryngeal cleft. Bronchoalveolar lavage fluid can be examined for fat-laden macrophages (**8.4**), suggestive, although not specifically, of aspiration (can also be seen in chronic bacterial infection).

High-resolution computed tomography scan

This may confirm the extent of the aspiration and rule out other diagnoses. Lower lobe disease commonly predominates (**8.5**).

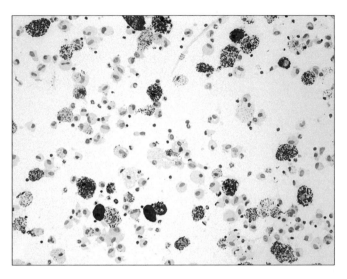

8.4 Histological slide from a bronchoalveolar lavage showing fat-laden macrophages (stained red).

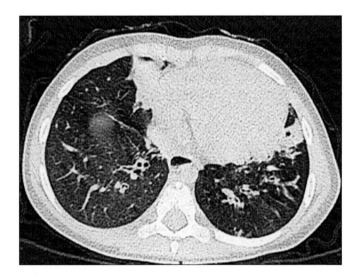

8.5 Computed tomography scan of the chest at the level of the lower lobes, showing bilateral bronchiectasis and areas of atelectasis secondary to gastro-oesophageal reflux and aspiration.

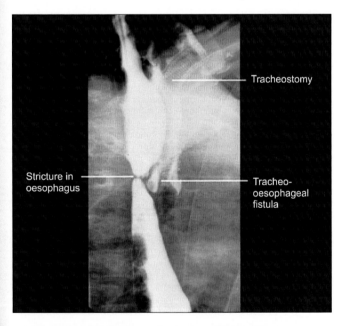

Tracheostomy

Stricture in oesophagus

Tracheo-oesophageal fistula

8.3 The tube oesophagram of a 2-year-old girl, with a tracheostomy. It shows a narrow stricture of the oesophagus at the level of the tip of the tracheostomy tube. At this site, a jet of contrast can be seen to pass from the oesophagus into the trachea, showing the presence of a tracheo-oesophageal fistula.

Gastro-oesophageal reflux

The investigations include:

- barium swallow
- milk scan
- 24-hour pH study
- multichannel intraluminal impedance study
- oesophagoscopy and biopsy.

Barium swallow

A barium swallow may confirm anatomical abnormalities such as a hiatus hernia, malrotation or pyloric stenosis. It is helpful in the study of swallowing, oesophageal motility, cardiac sphincter function, GOR (**8.6**) and gastric emptying during the awake period, and can also be useful in assessing if a fundoplication performed previously is still intact (**8.7**). However, both false negative and false positive results are common and the test is not often used in isolation.

Milk scan

This study may be used to complement the barium swallow. It is rarely associated with false negative results. It is performed by using a technetium 99m sulphur colloid mixed with a feed. Detectors are placed under the subject and the passage of the tagged meal is monitored from the oesophagus into the stomach as well as the transit time in the stomach. Reappearance of radioactivity in the oesophagus is indicative of GOR (**8.8**). Up to 3% of documented reflux

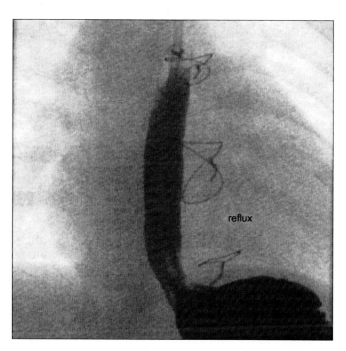

8.6 Barium swallow showing gastro-oesophageal reflux past the mid-oesophagus. This child had a ventricular septal defect repaired in the past and hence the presence of sternotomy wires.

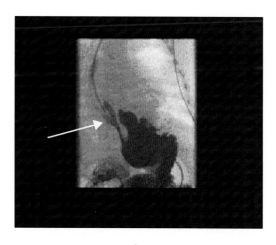

8.7 Barium study via the nasogastric tube of a 2-year-old boy with recurrent chest infections, who had had a Nissen's fundoplication performed aged 6 months. The Nissen's wrap is partially loosened and some of it appears above the level of the diaphragm. A moderate amount of reflux is also seen (indicated by the arrow).

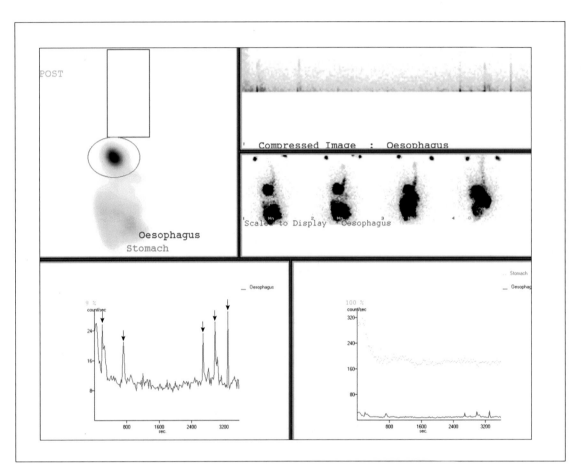

8.8 Milk scan demonstrating episodes of gastro-oesophageal reflux. The compressed images show at least five peaks of increased activity within the region of interest encompassing the oesophagus, suggesting five episodes of gastro-oesophageal reflux in the 1-hour study. This is highlighted in the time–activity curve by the black arrows.

is normal. Reappearance of radioactivity in the lung fields indicates reflux and aspiration.

24-hour pH study

The most widely accepted tool for the diagnosis of GOR is intra-oesophageal pH monitoring, which is used to measure the number and duration of acid reflux episodes during a 24-hour period. The test is performed by the placement of a microelectrode into the lower oesophagus. The ideal position of the sensor is between T8 and T10, confirmed by a chest radiograph (**8.9**). In infants, frequent milk feeds may neutralize gastric acid and the administration of alternative, non-alkaline feeds such as apple juice may be required. Alternatively, dual probes are now available, which simultaneously detect gastric acidity and calculate the reflux index on this basis.

Reflux and aspiration 87

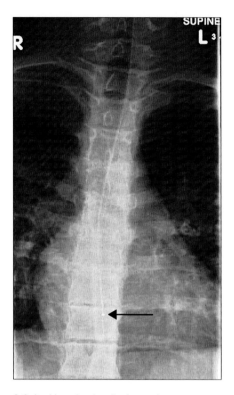

8.9 A pH probe *in situ* (arrow) as observed on a chest X-ray.

An episode of acid reflux is defined as an oesophageal pH of <4 for a specified minimum duration, usually 15–30 seconds. The data are reported as total time or percentage of the study time with pH <4; number of episodes of pH <4 in a 24-hour period; and the number of episodes lasting longer than 5 minutes (example in **8.10**).

The limitation of this method is that it does not document the reflux of non-acid fluid from the stomach into the oesophagus. Furthermore, in some patients, oesophageal pH monitoring may be within the normal range but brief episodes of GOR may cause complications of acute life-threatening episodes, cough or aspiration pneumonia.

Multichannel intraluminal impedance study
The multiple intraluminal electrical impedance technique (**8.11**) is a method for evaluating GOR based on the detection of gastrointestinal motility. The principle of this test is to measure the change of electrical impedance that occurs during the passage of a bolus between two adjacent electrodes. The use of multiple measuring segments along a catheter placed along the full length of the oesophagus allows analysis of the direction of the bolus transport. The

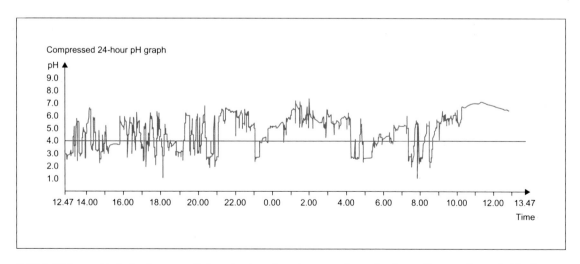

8.10 A 24-hour pH study shows multiple episodes of gastro-oesophageal reflux, with oesophageal pH <4.

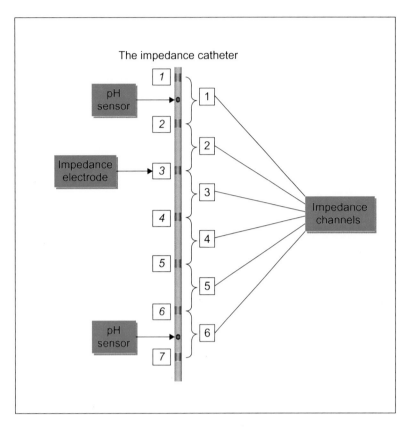

The impedance catheter

8.11 The impedance catheter and its components.

multichannel intraluminal impedance study has been shown to be a valuable tool for evaluating non-acid GOR; for distinguishing between anterograde and retrograde bolus movements; for assessing the height reached by the refluxate in the oesophagus; and for evaluating the clearance process of GOR. The simultaneous use of pH recording and the multiple intraluminal impedance technique increases the sensitivity of detecting reflux.

However, the multichannel intraluminal impedance study is currently not a routine clinical test and the absence of normative data is a significant limitation.

Oesophagoscopy and biopsy

These invasive tests are the only way to determine the presence and severity of oesophagitis (**8.12**). A normal macroscopic appearance does not exclude histopathological oesophagitis. Subtle mucosal changes such as erythema and pallor may be observed in the absence of oesophagitis and biopsy is therefore recommended.

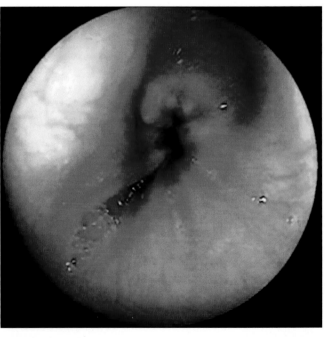

8.12 Macroscopic oesophagitis in a 5-year-old boy with cystic fibrosis who had a persistent cough despite maximal treatment with antibiotics and antireflux treatment.

Therapy and management

The medical and surgical treatment goals of aspiration and GOR are the same, i.e. relief of symptoms, mucosal healing, treatment and prevention of complications.

Aspiration from above

Depending on the aetiology, the management can involve repairing the anomaly causing the aspiration, e.g. tracheo-oesophageal fistula. However, in many cases where the aspiration is due to swallowing incoordination or weakness, joint management with a speech and language therapist is essential. Thickening the feeds may improve swallowing and reduce the risk of aspiration. In more severe cases, the only solution may be a nasogastric tube or gastrostomy.

Gastro-oesophageal reflux
Medical
Positioning

Prone positioning reduces GOR in infants, although this position is currently not recommended because of the increased risk of sudden infant death syndrome. Placing an infant in an infant car seat during and after feeding may reduce the frequency of GOR.

Thickened feeds

Milk thickening agents, such as rice cereal do not improve reflux index scores but do decrease the number of episodes of vomiting.

Pharmacology

The purpose of pharmacological agents such as H_2 receptor antagonists, proton pump inhibitors and prokinetic agents is to reduce the amount of acid refluxate to which the oesophagus or respiratory tract is exposed. The aim of acid suppressants is to decrease acid production. The prokinetic agents will reduce the amount of refluxate by improving contractility of the body of the oesophagus, increasing pressure in the lower oesophageal sphincter, decreasing the frequency of transient lower oesophageal sphincter relaxations and accelerating gastric emptying.

Histamine 2 receptor antagonists

These act to decrease acid secretion by inhibiting the H_2 receptor on the gastric parietal cell. Ranitidine is most commonly used in children in the UK, but cimetidine, famotidine and nizatidine are also used worldwide.

Proton pump inhibitors (PPIs)

PPIs covalently bond and deactivate the H^+, K^+, ATPase pumps and produce more sustained inhibition of acid secretion then H_2 receptor antagonists. PPIs include omeprazole, lansoprazole and pantoprazole. Specifically, omeprazole has been shown to be highly effective in the treatment of severe oesophagitis, resulting in both symptomatic and endoscopic improvement while on treatment. Optimal effectiveness is achieved when the PPI is administered 30 minutes before a meal so that peak plasma concentrations coincide with mealtimes. A steady state of acid suppression is not achieved for several days.

Prokinetic agents

The rationale for prokinetic agents such as domperidone, metoclopramide and cisapride in the treatment of GOR is based on evidence that they enhance oesophageal peristalsis and accelerate gastric emptying. Metoclopramide is an antidopaminergic agent with cholinomimetic and mixed serotonergic effects. Although the use of metoclopramide may decrease the frequency of vomiting, further data suggest frequent extrapyramidal side effects and there have been case reports of cardiac toxicity.

Domperidone is a peripheral antidopaminergic agent and does not readily cross the central nervous system. It increases motility and gastric emptying. As the marketing authorizations for cisapride were suspended in the UK in 2000 due to safety concerns, domperidone has been widely used by paediatricians to treat GOR. There are limited data on the efficacy of domperidone with only two randomized controlled trials reporting improvement in symptoms of GOR after treatment, with no noted adverse effects.

Erythromycin improves gastroduodenal prokinetic activity, although effectiveness may decrease over time.

Surgical

The surgical options of fundoplication include a Nissen's fundoplication (360° wrap), Thal fundoplication (210–270° wrap) and Toupet procedure (180° wrap). These procedures are not without complications, including failure, which necessitates re-operation in up to 20%. In the past, fundoplications were performed through a relatively large upper abdominal incision and required a long hospital stay, although they are now frequently being performed laparoscopically, with lower morbidity and shorter hospital stays.

Summary

Respiratory disease in children can not only contribute to, but also be caused by GOR and aspiration. The mechanisms by which GOR precipitates respiratory illness in children remain incompletely understood. The presentations of GOR and aspiration are highly variable and a complex set of investigations may be required to establish the diagnosis. Prompt diagnosis will allow early initiation of treatment, either medical and/or surgical, with the ultimate goal of limiting chronic respiratory disease.

Further reading

Euler AR, Byrne WJ. Twenty-four-hour esophageal intraluminal pH probe testing: a comparative analysis. *Gastroenterology* 1981; 80: 957–61.

Hyman PE. Gastroesophageal reflux: one reason why baby won't eat. *J Pediatr* 1994: 125: S103–9.

Kimber C, Kiely EM, Spitz L. The failure rate of surgery for gastro-oesophageal reflux. *J Pediatr Surg* 1998; 33: 64–6.

Loughlin GM, Lefton-Greif MA. Dysfunctional swallowing and respiratory disease in children. *Adv Pediatr* 1994; 41: 135–62.

Rudolph, CD, Mazur LJ, Liptak GS, *et al.* Guidelines for evaluation and treatment of gastroesophageal reflux in infants and children: recommendations of the North American Society for Pediatric Gastroenterology and Nutrition. *J Pediatr Gastroenterol Nutr* 2001; 32(Suppl 2):S1–31.

Chapter 9

The immunodeficient child

Andrew R. Gennery, David Anthony Spencer

Introduction

Humans have large surface area lungs, which are moist, warm and permeable, a welcoming environment for a wide variety of micro-organisms. To counter potentially fatal interactions with such organisms, protective mechanisms have evolved, which may sometimes fail. Immunodeficiency is often categorized by major and minor forms; however, functional immaturities of the system, which can only be assessed by monitoring changes in immune function over time, are more common. Recognition of both rare infections and unusual patterns of common infection suggestive of immunodeficiency reduces late diagnosis and the consequent excess morbidity and mortality. An understanding of the different immune mechanisms helps in the rational planning of investigations.

Immune defences

These can be broadly divided into barriers, first-line non-specific innate responses and second-line acquired or specific responses (*Table 9.1*). Innate immunity is characterized by cells and proteins that non-specifically recognize invading pathogens (*Table 9.2*). The magnitude of response is similar for each encounter. Macrophages link innate and specific acquired immune responses. The acquired system has memory, allowing greater and more rapid response each time the same antigen is encountered. This system consists of T-helper and T-cytotoxic lymphocytes, as well as B lymphocytes and plasma cells, which secrete immunoglobulin (*Table 9.3*). T and B lymphocytes that have encountered antigen can become long-lived memory cells that are primed to counter the same antigen if it is met again.

Congenital antibody deficiency

These are the commonest of the immunodeficiencies in patients with recurrent sinopulmonary infection. However, distinguishing patients with frequent infection but normal immunity from those with primary immunodeficiency can be difficult. It is considered normal for a child of up to 5 years of age to suffer eight to ten upper respiratory tract infections per year, typically with increased frequency of episodes in the winter months.

Specific warning signs of immunodeficiency include:

- more than one episode of proven pneumonia
- invasive infections in more than one system (e.g. pneumonia and meningitis)
- severe, unusual or persistent infections
- requirement of surgery for chronic infection, such as tonsillectomy, grommets or boil incision
- instigation of second-line tests for chronic infections (e.g. sweat tests or ciliary function tests)
- infections in patients with pre-existing autoimmune disease
- absent lymphoid tissue, e.g. absent thymic shadow, lack of peripheral lymph nodes
- unexplained signs, such as hepatosplenomegaly or arthropathy
- family history of primary immunodeficiency
- parental consanguinity.

Transient hypogammaglobulinaemia of infancy
Maternal IgG is actively transferred from mother to foetus during the third trimester of pregnancy, giving high immunoglobulin levels at birth that decay over the next

Table 9.1 Immune defences

Barrier	Innate immunity	Acquired (adaptive) immunity
Mechanical	Cellular	T lymphocytes
Epithelial cells and tight junctions	Phagocytes	CD4+ helper T cells
Longitudinal flow of air or fluid	Neutrophils	T_H1 cells
Movement of mucus by cilia	Basophils	T_H2 cells
Nasal barrier, impacting large particles	Eosinophils	CD8+ cytotoxic T cells
	Macrophages	
	Natural killer cells	
Chemical	Chemical	B lymphocytes
Fatty acids	Complement	Plasma cells – secrete immunoglobulin
Low pH	Mannose-binding lectin	
Enzymes	C-reactive protein	
Antibacterial peptides	Collectins	
Microbiological		Immunoglobulin
Normal flora		IgM
		IgA
		IgG1–4
		IgE

Table 9.2 Innate immunity

Component	Function	Receptors
Complement	Binds to micro-organisms	C3b binds covalently to pathogen
	Initiates inflammation	Mannose-binding lectin is a pattern-recognition receptor
	Recruits phagocytes	
	Opsonization	
	Enhances phagocytosis	
	Direct lysis of bacterial cell wall	
Neutrophils	Engulf and destroy micro-organisms	Germline-encoded phagocyte receptors recognize pathogens directly, through pattern-recognition receptors
	Phagocytosis aided by complement and antibody receptors	
Macrophages	Engulf micro-organisms	Pattern-recognition receptor
	Process engulfed pathogens and break them down into peptides	Toll-like receptors
	Present peptides in association with major histocompatibility complex class I or II molecules to T lymphocytes	Induce inflammatory cytokines
		Cause upregulation of co-stimulatory molecules on macrophages, dendritic cells, T cells

Table 9.3 Adaptive immunity

Component	Function	Receptors
CD4+ T$_H$1 cell	Activates macrophages to destroy intracellular pathogens, e.g. *Mycobacterium tuberculosis*	T-cell receptor
CD4+ T$_H$2 cell	Activates B cells to produce immunoglobulin	T-cell receptor
CD4+ T cell	Activates CD8+ T cells	T-cell receptor
CD8+ T cell	Destroys virally infected nucleated cells	T-cell receptor
CD19+ B cell	Produces immunoglobulin (IgM, IgA, IgG, IgE), which bind extracellular pathogens and aid phagocytosis	B-cell receptor

4–6 months. As the infant encounters antigenic stimuli, it begins to make antibody, initially IgM then switching to IgG. Intrinsic IgG production may be delayed, so as transferred maternal IgG levels fall through natural decay, a transient IgG nadir occurs between 4 and 6 months that may be associated with a predisposition to infection. IgG levels generally normalize by 12 months of age but the physiological nadir may occasionally be prolonged for up to 2 years. Transient hypogammaglobulinaemia of infancy is a retrospective diagnosis.

Polysaccharide antibody deficiency

Encapsulated bacterial polysaccharide antibody deficiency is one of the most common presentations to paediatric immunology clinics. Pneumococcal polysaccharide antibody deficiency is the most characteristic problem, and is the easiest to assess, but if children cannot respond to pneumococcal antigen, they are also likely to fail to respond to the capsular antigens of other bacteria. Below 2 years of age, most children cannot make antibody against bacterial polysaccharide. Children under 5 years may have a delay in making polysaccharide antibody and may present with recurrent pulmonary infections partially because of close contact with other children in nurseries. These patients also fail to respond adequately to pneumococcal polysaccharide vaccine. In those with polysaccharide antibody maturational delay, the prognosis is good; by 5–6 years of age they make pneumococcal polysaccharide antibody and infections become less frequent. In a minority of patients this defect may be a manifestation of other underlying combined immunodeficiencies, such as DiGeorge syndrome or Wiskott–Aldrich syndrome, and other

features characteristic of these diseases should be sought (*Table 9.4*). Maturational antibody delay is a retrospective diagnosis, often associated with low serum concentrations of IgG2 and IgA.

Common variable immune deficiency

Common variable immune deficiency, classically a disease of late adolescence and early-to-middle adulthood, is increasingly diagnosed in young children. It is a poorly characterized condition although recognized features include low levels of two or more major antibody isotypes, impaired specific antibody responses and sometimes T-lymphocyte impairment. The main clinical presentation is recurrent pulmonary infection with organisms such as *Haemophilus influenzae* and *Streptococcus pneumoniae*. Bronchiectasis is inevitable if diagnosis or treatment are delayed. It is important to exclude other known genetic causes of immunodeficiency before giving a label of common variable immune deficiency to a young child.

Primary agammaglobulinaemia

Several genetic defects lead to absence of one or more major classes of antibody. X-linked agammaglobulinaemia (Bruton's disease) is the best characterized, but autosomal recessive forms are described. Cardinal features of primary antibody deficiency are the same regardless of the underlying genetic defect:

- symptoms begin between 6 and 12 months of age as maternally acquired IgG decays;

Table 9.4 Combined immunodeficiencies

Syndrome	Genetic defect	Clinical features
DiGeorge syndrome	Heterozygous 22q11.2 deletion Rarely chromosome 10p deletion	Classic facies (hypertelorism, antimongoloid slant of eyes, broad nasal bridge, long philtrum, posteriorly rotated ear with simple helix, bulbous nose tip, micrognathia) Cardiac defect (classically truncus arteriosus or interrupted aortic arch, but others described) Hypoparathyroidism Immunodeficiency, rarely SCID, more commonly antibody deficiency
Wiskott–Aldrich syndrome	Wiskott–Aldrich syndrome protein (*WAS*) Xp11.4–p11.21	Eczema, Thrombocytopenia with reduced platelet volume (<5 fl) Recurrent infection Epstein–Barr virus associated lymphoreticular malignancy
CD40 ligand deficiency	CD40 ligand (CD154) Xq26	*Pneumocystis jiroveci* (previously *carinii*) pneumonia Recurrent bacterial pneumonia Oral ulceration Cryptosporidial diarrhoea
Ataxia telangiectasia	Ataxia telangiectasia mutated (*ATM*) 11q22–q23	Progressive cerebellar ataxia Oculocutaneous telangiectasia (usually not present until >2 years old) Recurrent sinopulmonary infection Lymphoid tumours
X-linked lymphoproliferative disease	SLAM-associated protein (*SH2D1A*) Xq25-q26	Fulminant Epstein–Barr viral infection Epstein–Barr virus associated lymphoreticular malignancy Hypogammaglobulinaemia with recurrent sinopulmonary infection

- chronic respiratory infection is the first manifestation in <70%;
- invasive bacterial infections in gastrointestinal tract or skin;
- diagnosis often delayed until 2.5–3.5 years of age or later.

Diagnostic delay often leads to chronic respiratory infection and bronchiectasis, which is the commonest cause of death in these patients. Patients presenting with recurrent invasive bacterial infection in the first year of life should be suspected of having an immunoglobulin deficiency until this has been excluded.

Combined immunodeficiencies and lung disease

Severe combined immunodeficiency

Severe combined immunodeficiency (SCID) involves T- and B-lymphocyte failure, and without treatment is generally fatal by 1 year of age. Different molecular defects give rise to a clinical picture of SCID (*Table 9.5*), but presenting features are common to all (*Table 9.6*). First hospitalization is generally between 45 and 100 days, affected infants presenting with an unremitting bronchiolitic illness of variable severity. Those with *Pneumocystis jiroveci* (previously *carinii*) pneumonia

(PJP) have a characteristic brassy cough and insidiously develop an oxygen requirement. Chest radiographs typically show patchy interstitial shadowing with hyperinflation (**9.1**), although almost any radiographic change may occur. Characteristically, the thymic shadow is absent and the midline pleural borders of the upper lobes may be visible (**9.2**). Patients with adenosine deaminase-deficient SCID may have characteristic skeletal abnormalities (**9.3**). Importantly, the differential white cell count may be diagnostic with a lymphopenia of $<2.8\times10^9/l$. Very rarely, patients may present with haemophagocytosis, or undifferentiated lymphoid malignancy, presumably because of lack of control from immunocompetent lymphocytes (**9.4**); such patients can be successfully treated with an infusion of replete marrow.

Table 9.5 Classification of severe combined immunodeficiency

Syndrome	T lymphocytes	B lymphocytes	NK lymphocytes	Inheritance
Reticular dysgenesis	–	–	–	AR
ADA deficiency	–	–	–	AR
RAG1, 2 deficiency	–	–	+	AR
Artemis deficiency (RS*)	–	–	+	AR
CgC deficiency	–	+	–	XL
JAK-3 deficiency	–	+	–	AR
IL-7Ra deficiency	–	+	+	AR
ZAP-70 kinase deficiency	CD4+	+	+	AR
MHC II deficiency	CD8+	+	+	AR
CD45 deficiency	+	+	+	AR

ADA, adenosine deaminase; AR, autosomal recessive; CgC, common interleukin γ chain; IL-7Ra, interleukin 7 receptor α; JAK-3, janus-associated kinase 3; RAG, recombination activating genes; XL, X-linked; ZAP-70, zeta-associated kinase-70.

Table 9.6 Presenting features of severe combined immunodeficiency

Common presentations	Common pathogens	Rare presentations
Persistent viral gastroenteritis	Norovirus	Bacterial septicaemia
	Rotavirus	
	Astrovirus	Disseminated BCG infection
	Adenovirus	
Persistent viral lower respiratory tract infection	Respiratory syncitial virus	Haemophagocytosis
Pneumocystis jiroveci pneumonitis	Parainfluenzae virus	
Recurrent or recalcitrant candidiasis	Cytomegalovirus	Lymphoid malignancy
Failure to thrive		Autoimmune cytopenias

BCG, Bacillus Calmette-Guérin.

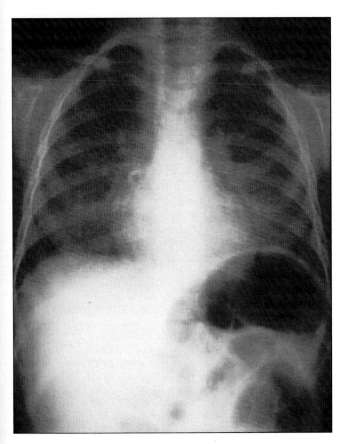

9.1 Chest radiograph from a 6-month-old infant presenting with an 8-week history of dry cough, increasing tachypnoea, and an evolving hypoxia. There is bilateral patchy shadowing typical of interstitial pneumonitis secondary to infection with respiratory viruses or *Pneumocystis jiroveci*.

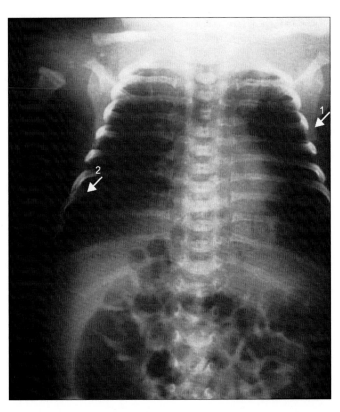

9.3 Chest radiograph from a 10-week-old infant with adenosine deaminase-deficient severe combined immunodeficiency showing abnormal scapulae (arrow 1) and cupping deformities of the ends of the ribs (arrow 2) – other abnormalities affect transverse vertebral processes.

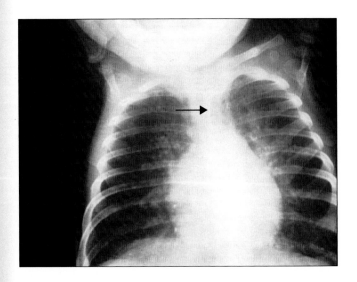

9.2 Chest radiograph from a 5-month-old infant with severe combined immunodeficiency, showing bilateral patchy shadowing secondary to interstitial pneumonitis due to infection with respiratory syncitial virus and *Pneumocystis jiroveci*. There is hyperinflation of the lungs and the mid-line pleural borders of the upper lobes are visible (arrowed) because the thymic shadow is absent.

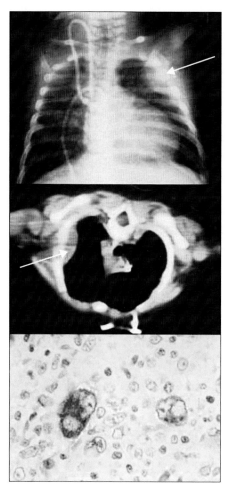

9.4 Undifferentiated lymphoid malignancy in a 7-month-old infant with severe combined immunodeficiency. A discrete shadow at the left upper lobe margin is seen on a plain chest radiograph (arrowed), and on computed tomography (arrowed). Tissue biopsy demonstrates an infiltrate of large uni- and bi-nucleated T cells and Reed–Sternberg-like cells (stained brown). The lesion resolved with a single dose of vincristine and an infusion of replete marrow.

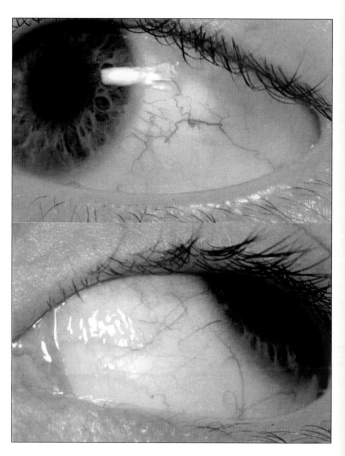

9.5 Ocular telangiectasia in a patient with ataxia-telangiectasia. Tortuous dilated blood vessels on the bulbar conjunctivae are typical findings, and often the first site of telangiectasia.

Other combined immunodeficiencies

Other combined immunodeficiencies with defects in T- and B-lymphocyte function present after infancy but are associated with a poor outcome in the longer term. Respiratory symptoms are common, usually secondary to hypogammaglobulinaemia or poor polysaccharide antibody responses. While specific defects may have characteristic presentations (*Table 9.4*; **9.5**), the respiratory presentations are rarely specific to a particular condition.

Phagocyte deficiencies

Phagocyte defects can lead to recurrent lung disease. Fungal infection is a particular risk in patients with neutropenia or non-functional neutrophils.

Chronic granulomatous disease

X-linked recessive inheritance is the commonest form of this disease, although autosomal forms are recognized. Acute suppurative lymphadenitis is a common manifestation but severe pneumonia may be the first sign of disease. Infections with organisms such as *Staphylococcus aureus*, *Burkholderia cepacia* complex and *Aspergillus* species are particularly common. Fungal infection often manifests as pneumonia, but disseminated infection frequently occurs, with osteomyelitis and hepatic involvement. Established fungal infection is hard to treat and frequently fatal. Non-infectious inflammatory sequelae are increasingly recognized, including restrictive lung defects. The defect lies in the phagocyte nicotinamide adenine dinucleotide phosphate oxidase enzyme complex (one component of which is inherited in an X-linked manner, the other three of which have autosomal recessive inheritance), which normally generates superoxide that is toxic to organisms ingested into phagosomes.

Hyper IgE syndrome (Job's syndrome)

Hyper IgE syndrome is characterized by extremely raised serum IgE (>400 units/litre, often several thousand units/litre), chronic dermatitis and repeated lung and skin infection. The classical presentation is *Staphylococcus aureus* pneumonia complicated by pneumatocoele formation, although infection with other organisms, including *Pseudomonas aeruginosa*, is recognized. Patients may develop chronic lung disease related to pneumatocoeles and bronchiectasis. Secondary aspergillus infection within old pneumatocoeles, causing an aspergillus mycetoma, is well recognized. The underlying defect in this condition has recently been identified.

Interferon-γ /interleukin 12 pathway defects

Defects in the interleukin-12-dependent interferon-γ pathway have been described in patients infected with poorly pathogenic environmental non-tuberculous mycobacteria (**9.6**); the infections are characteristically severe, persistent and invasive, occurring in bone and soft tissue abscesses or disseminated throughout the body, and are often fatal. An increased susceptibility to viral infection including human herpes viruses, and respiratory viruses including respiratory syncitial virus and parainfluenzae viruses, is also described. Infections result from a failure of upregulation of macrophage killing.

Primary inherited complement deficiencies

Severe disease due to complement deficiencies is inherited in an autosomal recessive manner with absolute deficiency of a complement component due to gene defects in both alleles. Heterozygosity with half normal protein levels may also be clinically important. Recurrent pyogenic infections are characteristic, with organisms such as streptococci and *Haemophilus influenzae* as the main pathogens because opsonization/binding of antibody and complement to bacteria is critical for their elimination. C3 deficiency is the most severe, but deficiency of the classical pathway components C1q and C2 and of factor D in the alternative pathway also predispose to infection. Deficiencies of the alternative pathway control proteins, factors H or I, lead to uncontrolled consumption of C3 resulting in increased susceptibility to pyogenic infections. Mannose-binding lectin (MBL) is a serum protein that binds to saccharides on bacterial cell walls resulting in cell death via complement activation. MBL deficiency is common, affecting up to 5% of the population. Numerous studies have associated MBL deficiency with an increased risk of infection. This defect is more relevant if there is an increased risk of infection in those with immature or ineffective adaptive immunity, for instance, with an associated antibody deficiency or having received chemotherapy.

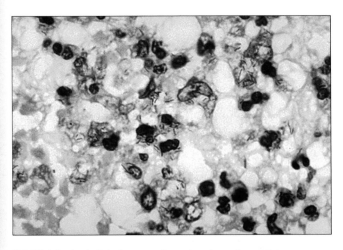

9.6 Histological stain from post mortem lung tissue taken from an 18-month-old child with a defect in the interleukin-12/interferon-γ pathway. Numerous pink rods of *Mycobacterium kansasii* are easily identified – there is no evidence of granuloma formation, the absence of which is characteristic of severe defects in the interleukin-12/interferon-γ pathway.

Secondary immunodeficiency

Secondary immunodeficiency states are increasingly encountered (*Table 9.7*). However, the immunodeficiency may be overlooked when focusing on the disease for which immunosuppression is being given. Improved treatment of malignancy, and organ and bone marrow transplantation now results in many more children receiving immunosuppressive drugs and radiotherapy. Immunity may also be compromised by immunoglobulin deficiency secondary to gastrointestinal protein loss or by complement consumption states.

Investigation of the child with recurrent or persistent pulmonary infection

Identifying which infectious agents are present will help predict the most likely deficiency in the immune system (*Table 9.8*). Children presenting with recurrent endobronchial infection or other warning signs of immunodeficiency require investigation (*Table 9.9*). Clinical features and radiographic findings are rarely diagnostic for specific infections. Often there are few clinical chest signs, yet widespread opacity

Table 9.7 Causes of secondary immunodeficiency

Secondary immunodeficiency

Infection
  Viral, including HIV
  Mycobacterial
Drugs
  Monoclonal antibodies
  Calcineurin antagonists
  Cytotoxic drugs
  Steroids
  Others
Radiotherapy
Haematopoietic stem cell transplantation
Solid organ transplantation
Protein-losing states
Hyposplenism
Malnutrition

Table 9.8 Primary immunodeficiencies and associated infections

Immunodeficiency	Causes	Commonly associated infection
T-cell immunodeficiency	Congenital combined immunodeficiency Chemotherapy Haematopoietic stem cell transplantation Solid organ transplantation	*Pneumocystis jiroveci*, respiratory syncytial virus, parainfluenza, cytomegalovirus, Epstein–Barr virus, adenoviruses
Antibody deficiency	Congenital antibody deficiency Antibody-losing state Chemotherapy Haematopoietic stem cell transplantation	*Streptococcus pneumoniae*, *Haemophilus influenzae*, other encapsulated bacteria, *Pseudomonas*, enteroviruses
Phagocyte defects	Congenital neutropenia Congenital neutrophil dysfunction Aplastic anaemia Haematopoietic stem cell transplantation (interferon γ/interleukin-12 defects)	*Streptococcus pneumoniae*, *Staphylococcus aureus*, *Pseudomonas*, *Burkholderia cepacia* complex, *Aspergillus*, *Nocardia* (atypical mycobacteria)
Complement deficiencies	Congenital deficiency	*Streptococcus pneumoniae*, *Meningococcus*, *Haemophilus* infection B

Table 9.9 Investigations in children with respiratory infection and suspected primary immunodeficiency	
First-line investigation	**Second-line investigation**
FBC and WCC differential	Chromosomal studies
Lymphocyte subsets	Genetic studies
IgM, A, G and IgG subclasses	HRCT of chest
Specific tetanus, HiB antibodies	Bronchoscopy
Pneumococcal antibodies (if >2 years)	Tissue biopsy
Simple spirometry (if >5 years)	Radiation sensitivity studies
Plain chest radiograph	Specific lymphocyte marker studies
Bronchoscopy	Lymphocyte proliferation investigations
Microbiological investigations (culture, IF, PCR)	Neutrophil oxidative burst investigations
Complement C3, C4, MBL levels	
Functional complement investigations	

C3,4, complement C3,4; FBC, full blood count; HiB, *Haemophilus influenzae* type B; HRCT, high-resolution computed tomography; IF, immunofluorescence; MBL, mannose-binding lectin; PCR, polymerase chain reaction; WCC, white cell count.

in the chest radiograph (**9.7**). Marked tachypnoea, few or no adventitial sounds on chest auscultation and a ground-glass appearance on the chest radiograph suggest interstitial pneumonitis; possible causes include PJP, cytomegalovirus and *Aspergillus*. Insidiously progressive respiratory deterioration with an oxygen requirement is more suggestive of PJP. When a child presents with pneumonitis a careful history is important, including:

- recent contact with individuals with known infection;
- contact with building work (increased risk of *Aspergillus* infection);
- recent travel.

Age-related reference ranges for immunoglobulins and lymphocyte numbers should be used as normal levels change with age; erroneous diagnosis may be made if adult reference ranges are used. Antibody deficiency to specific antigens, commonly pneumococcal polysaccharide antigens, can occur despite normal levels of IgG and IgG subclasses. It is normal for infants in the first 2–3 years of life to respond poorly to polysaccharide antigens. Low specific antibody levels should be rechecked 4 weeks following vaccination challenge (a less than four-fold rise in antibody level to within the normal range is abnormal). Other abnormalities

require further investigation or a search for specific genetic defects. IgA and IgG$_2$ subclass deficiency are commonly inconsequential. Isolated low IgA levels in an asymptomatic child require no further investigation or treatment, but true IgA absence should be determined by the Ouchterlony test, as complete absence may presage recurrent infection or autoimmunity.

All children with suspected immunodeficiency should have a detailed respiratory assessment. A plain chest radiograph is important, but may be completely normal. High-resolution computerized tomography of the chest is frequently necessary and can be particularly helpful in revealing bronchiectasis. Characteristic changes are also found in patients with invasive aspergillosis where nodules or areas of consolidation may be surrounded by a halo of ground-glass opacity. Spirometry can usually be performed from 5 years of age; although single measures have little diagnostic value, serial measurements may give an early warning of respiratory deterioration.

More invasive procedures to obtain respiratory secretions or lung tissue may be needed; bronchoalveolar lavage should be considered early. Computed tomography is useful to locate the site of infected lung tissue when tissue sampling is required to make the diagnosis. Computed tomography-guided percutaneous needle aspiration may be a useful

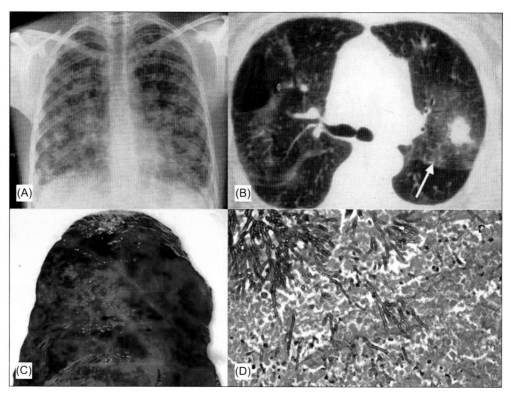

9.7 (A) Chest radiograph of a 15-year-old boy with autosomal recessive chronic granulomatous disease, showing bilateral dense infiltrates. (B) Computed tomography demonstrates a pulmonary nodule surrounded by a zone of ground-glass attenuation (arrowed), features highly suggestive of angioinvasive fungal infection, most commonly *Aspergillus* species. (C) At post mortem, the lung was solid and haemorrhagic with discrete areas of necrosis. (D) Histological examination showed characteristic branching hyphae of aspergillus. *Aspergillus fumigatus* and *Absidia corymbifera* were grown from post mortem culture specimens.

way to obtain diagnostic material for the identification of specific micro-organisms such as *Mycobacterium tuberculosis*, *Staphylococcus aureus*, *Aspergillus fumigatus* and *Cryptococcus neoformans*. However, an open lung biopsy may be necessary if a causative organism is not isolated by this investigation (**9.8**); this is to be preferred to the performance of repeated bronchoalveolar lavages. Specimens of sputum, blood and nasopharyngeal secretions should be sent for bacteriological and virological examination. Careful liaison with laboratory staff is important if the correct samples are to be obtained and the correct investigations performed. Serology is unhelpful in antibody-deficient states. Upper respiratory tract specimens obtained from nasal washes, nasopharyngeal aspirates or nasopharyngeal swabs are usually better than throat swabs but can be difficult to obtain in young children.

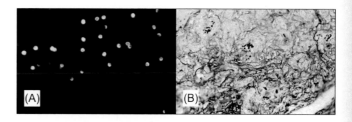

9.8 *Pneumocystis jiroveci* demonstrated by (A) immunofluorescence on a bronchoalveolar lavage specimen, and (B) silver staining of alveolar tissue from a lung biopsy.

Treatment of immunodeficiency

Patients with mild or transient defects in the ability to manufacture antibodies against encapsulated bacteria can often be managed successfully with antibiotics. These may need to be given intermittently or continuously according to the clinical situation, and frequently at higher doses than used in immunocompetent children. In severe antibody deficiency, immunoglobulin replacement, supervised by a paediatric immunologist, is required. Importantly, immunoglobulin is a blood product with the potential to transmit infections such as hepatitis C. Before instituting treatment it should be ascertained by polymerase chain reaction that there is no previous infection with hepatitis C. Spirometry should be performed, at least annually, and high-resolution computed tomography performed biannually. Patients with complement deficiencies should be treated with broad-spectrum prophylactic antibiotics such as co-trimoxazole.

Severe T-cell and phagocyte deficiencies can be cured by haematopoietic stem cell transplantation, but the prognosis may be significantly compromised by pre-existing lung damage.

Close liaison between the respiratory paediatrician and immunologist is essential and we suggest that each regional centre should establish a joint respiratory/immunology clinic for the management of these complex patients.

Conclusions

Recurrent pulmonary infection is common in childhood, and for a minority of children is the presentation of immunodeficiency. An awareness of unusual patterns of presentation and the warning signs of immunodeficiency will alert the clinician to the possibility of an underlying defect, leading to appropriate investigation and treatment. Earlier recognition of these rare conditions will prevent the development of life-threatening sequelae.

Acknowledgements

All photographs are supplied courtesy of the Paediatric Immunology Unit, Newcastle General Hospital.

Further reading

Cant AJ, Gibb D, Davies EG, Cale C, Gennery AR. Immunodeficiency. In: *Forfar and Arneil's Textbook of Pediatrics*, 7th edn. McIntosh N, Helms P, Smyth R (eds). Edinburgh: Churchill Livingstone, 2008: pp. 1139–76.

Casanova JL, Abel L. Genetic dissection of immunity to mycobacteria: the human model. *Annu Rev Immunol* 2002; 20: 581–620.

Gennery AR, Cant AJ. Respiratory infection in the immunocompromised host: recognition and treatment. In: *The Microbe-Host Interface in Respiratory Tract Infections*. Kimpen JLL, Ramilo O (eds). Wymondham, UK: Horizon Scientific Press Ltd, 2005: pp. 47–94.

Gennery AR, Spencer DA, Cant AJ. Immune deficiency and the lung. *Curr Paediatr* 2004; 14: 115–21.

Klein NJ. Mannose-binding lectin: do we need it? *Mol Immunol* 2005; 42: 919–24.

Index

Note: page numbers in *italics* refer to Figures and Tables.